T0319548

A Research Agenda for Disability and Technology

Elgar Research Agendas outline the future of research in a given area. Leading scholars are given the space to explore their subject in provocative ways, and map out the potential directions of travel. They are relevant but also visionary.

Forward-looking and innovative, Elgar Research Agendas are an essential resource for PhD students, scholars and anybody who wants to be at the forefront of research.

For a full list of Edward Elgar published titles, including the titles in this series, visit our website at www.e-elgar.com

A Research Agenda for Disability and Technology

Edited by

JANE SEALE

Professor of Education, Faculty of Wellbeing, Education and Language Studies, The Open University, UK

Elgar Research Agendas

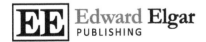 Edward Elgar
PUBLISHING

Cheltenham, UK • Northampton, MA, USA

Published by
Edward Elgar Publishing Limited
The Lypiatts
15 Lansdown Road
Cheltenham
Glos GL50 2JA
UK

Edward Elgar Publishing, Inc.
William Pratt House
9 Dewey Court
Northampton
Massachusetts 01060
USA

A catalogue record for this book
is available from the British Library

Library of Congress Control Number: 2024930471

This book is available electronically in the **Elgar**online
Sociology, Social Policy and Education subject collection
http://dx.doi.org/10.4337/9781800888647

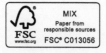

ISBN 978 1 80088 863 0 (cased)
ISBN 978 1 80088 864 7 (eBook)

Printed and bound in Great Britain by
TJ Books Limited, Padstow, Cornwall

Contents

Figures

Tables

Contributors

Shamima Akhtar is an accessibility policy expert specialising in employment, education, accessible transport, digital inclusion and independent living policy. She supports the All-Party Parliamentary Group for Assistive Technology, the ATech Policy Lab and the Higher Education Commission at Policy Connect.

Huseyin Dogan is a Professor of Human Computer Interaction at the University of Bournemouth, UK, where he is Co-founder and Co-chair of the Human Computer Interaction (HCI) research group. His research focuses on human factors, assistive technology, digital health and systems engineering. He has eight years' industrial experience working as a Higher Scientist for BAE Systems Advanced Technology Centre.

Dave Edyburn is a Senior Research Scientist and Professor Emeritus at the University of Wisconsin, Milwaukee, US. His research and teaching interests focus on the use of technology to enhance teaching, learning and performance; the nexus of human and machine learning; special education technology research; and universal design for learning. He has authored over 175 articles and book chapters on the use of technology in special education. His work represents a variety of contributions to theory, research and practice.

Alan Foley is an Associate Professor in the Department of Cultural Foundations of Education at Syracuse University, US, and coordinates the Disability Studies Program there. His research explores constructions of disability, technology and access, and he is currently engaged in participatory research projects on access to community living and participation via mobile technology. He has authored book chapters, white papers and technical reports on educational technology and assistive technology.

Clive Gilbert leads the Assistive and Accessible Technology Team's social care and independent living and industry and innovation policy workstreams at Policy Connect. He is a member of the UK government's Digital Social Care Advisory Group and a member of the governing council of the British Assistive Technology Association (BATA).

Tom Griffiths is a Lecturer in Assistive Technology at the University of Dundee, UK, and a state-registered Clinical Scientist, who has previously held the role of Assistive Technologist in an NHS Specialist AAC service. Tom has a clinical and research interest in the use of eye-gaze technology by children with cerebral palsy. This connects to a broader interest in access to computers and assistive technology for people with disabilities and increasing participation through provision of technology.

J. Bern Jordan is a Researcher in the College of Information Studies at the University of Maryland and Director of the Rehabilitation Engineering Research Center on ICT Access (previously the Trace RERC). His work includes the development of techniques for cross-disability access to public ICT, the development of cross-disability user experiences, analysis of and contributions to accessibility standards and regulations, the development of hands-on accessibility training workshops, and research into automatically generating personal, one-size-fits-one interfaces, and open-source photosensitive epilepsy analysis tools.

Crystal Marte is a Program Associate at the nonprofit organisation 'Raising the Floor'. At the Trace Center, she has conducted accessibility research spanning multiple areas, including Artificial Intelligence fairness, older adults and people with dementia and their technology use and emerging mainstream and assistive technologies.

Robert McLaren is the Director of Policy Connect's ATech Policy Lab in the UK which brings together disabled people, researchers and the tech sector to design evidence-based policy to make technology work for everyone. Robert authored two reports while at Policy Connect, *Accessible VLEs* (2018) and *Disabled Students' Allowances* (2019). Robert chairs the Department for Education's Assistive Technology Engagement Group and is a Senior Policy Fellow (Technology) at the Disability Policy Centre.

Jane Seale is a Professor of Education at the Open University, UK. Between 2000 and 2002 Jane set up the first ever UK-based Masters in Assistive Technology at Kings College, London. A major area of her research focuses on the role that technologies play in the lives of people with learning disabilities. For example during the pandemic she examined whether and how people with learning disabilities were being supported to use technologies to keep connected and stay well.

Rohan Slaughter is a Senior Lecturer in Assistive Technology at the University of Dundee, UK. Rohan is a teacher, Assistive Technologist and specialist education leader and has over 20 years' experience of supporting access to technology in the education sector. He has conducted practically focused research projects such as the Dart project, Connect to Control and the BT-funded Wheeltop project. This experience base covers assistive technology, educational leadership and IT infrastructure.

Gregg Vanderheiden is the founder and Director Emeritus of the Trace R&D Center in the US and a Professor in the College of Information Studies at the University of Maryland. He is a pioneer in the field of augmentative communication, assistive technology and computer access. Access features developed by Gregg and the Trace Center team can be found in every computer and mobile device internationally. He created the first Web Content Accessibility Guidelines (WCAG) in 1995 and co-chaired the Working Group for WCAG 1 and 2.

Annalu Waller is a Professor of Human Communication Technologies at the University of Dundee, UK, where she directs the Dundee AT/AAC Research Group. Annalu has worked in the field of augmentative and alternative communication (AAC) since 1985, designing communication systems for and with non-speaking individuals. Her primary research areas are human computer interaction, natural language processing, personal narrative and assistive technology. In particular, she focuses on empowering end users and has pioneered the inclusion of people with complex disabilities in research and teaching.

Paul Whittington is a Lecturer in Assistive Technology in the Faculty of Science & Technology at Bournemouth University. His research focuses on assistive technologies, human factors, usability engineering and system of systems. He is a member of the Human Computer Interaction (HCI) Research Group and teaches on the BSc Human Factors in Computing Systems and MSc Human Factors units.

Preface

The focus of this book is researching the relationship between disability and assistive technology (AT). AT (sometimes called assistive products[1,2]) can be non-digital (e.g., prosthetic leg) or digital (e.g., electronic communication aid); low tech (e.g., walking cane) or high tech (e.g., environmental control systems). For the purposes of this book, we will predominantly focus on digital technologies (hereafter referred to interchangeably either as technology or assistive technology). Assistive technology will be broadly defined as including computers (desktop, laptops); mobile phones including smartphones and all the apps that can be used on them; personal digital assistants and other tablet devices; the Internet and email; social media; electronic communication aids; telecare equipment; environmental control systems; virtual and augmented reality systems; games consoles and associated games; and robots and artificial intelligence systems.

The contributors to the book are drawn from the disability and technology community and represent a range of different stakeholders including researchers, developers, policy professionals, practitioners and people with disabilities. Although they are based in the United Kingdom and the United States of America, in writing their chapters, they have drawn extensively on international literature spanning both the Global North and the Global South.

The primary readership for the book is postgraduate students and researchers in the fields of assistive technology, computer science, human–computer interaction, rehabilitation science/engineering, art and design, critical disability studies, science and technology studies, occupational therapy, medicine, speech and language therapy, nursing, social work, social policy, law and education. With this in mind, the book has drawn on a wide range of research, policy and practice literature.

A significant proportion of the literature in the disability and technology research community adopts an overarching master narrative that positions technology as having incredible potential to transform the lives of people with disabilities (Seale, 2020). Alongside this narrative, there can be an assumption that the needs and difficulties of people with disabilities are so great that only 'high-tech', state-of-the-art technologies will bring about the necessary transformation. This narrative has often been reinforced when the community is able to point to high-profile examples of people with disabilities whose success in their field is perceived to be due in whole or in part to their use of 'high-tech' technologies. A classic example is the award-winning astrophysicist, Professor Stephen Hawking, who became paralysed as a consequence of developing motor neurone disease and famously used a computer-based communication aid and a powered wheelchair. In a research project focused on the history of technology use, I interviewed 52 professionals who had worked in the special educational needs field for ten years or more about their memories and experiences (Seale, 2019). Several of the professionals shared how, in talking to parents and children with special educational needs about the potential of technology and what it could do for them, they had often used Stephen Hawking as an example or role model:

> I used the example of Stephen Hawking when I was trying to explain to people, the sort of work I did. Especially in France where people understand very little about disability, let alone technology. And they all know Stephen Hawking and so he is a very good role model. (Teacher and Advisor)
>   When I say to people, I have been working with people who use switches to communicate – I will tend to say – you know, like Stephen Hawking, because they know that physically he is very limited and yet he is able to speak through his computer. So I use him to encapsulate the whole notion of technology allowing you to communicate when you physically can't. (Developer)

Such a narrative and its underpinning assumptions about the power of technology to overcome the deficits of people with disabilities has advantages, particularly in relation to persuading research agencies to fund new research and development projects. However, it also has disadvantages, which I suggest need to be considered in any proposals for a future research agenda. Firstly, it can lead to unrealistic expectations regarding the potential impact or success of technologies. For example, in my study, those practitioners who invoked Stephen Hawking as a role model were acutely aware that it might give parents and disabled children unrealistic expectations of what they could achieve through their technology use:

> Like parents who see Stephen Hawking and say – I want Stephen Hawking's kit for my kid. If I have that for my child, it will work. No, it won't work! Because your little one is 3 or 4 years old, they need something more akin to them and they can have fun and they can grow and then we can add things on. They might end up with that. But that was a hard argument with lots of parents and also with teaching staff.

That you need what is appropriate to the person at the time – not where you hope they will get to – because there might be an awful lot of steps before they get there. (Speech Therapist and Advisor)

I am hoping that people will understand that the majority of people are not at [Stephen Hawking's] intellectual level, it is just that that is an example of technology in action [...] there is a danger in having him as a role model that people will assume the output that you generate is going to be at [his] level of fluency. That would be wrong. (Developer)

In 2001, John Hockenberry, who was a news correspondent with Dateline NBC at the time, gave a keynote speech in which he shared his experiences of using technologies following an accident that resulted in him being paraplegic.[3] Through his interactions with able-bodied friends, family and colleagues regarding the potential of technology, he experienced what he called 'two competing mythologies'. The first was that all assistive technology is advanced and magical and the second was that massively ambitious goals are the only ones that are worth striving to achieve through the use of technology:

I was trying to figure out what the deal was, what capabilities were going to be available to me, given that I was going back to college, what would be the consequences of my loss of functioning [...] A family friend said to me, you know, John, what you need is a jetpack [...] when you are a paraplegic and in a wheelchair and somebody says to you, what you need is a jetpack, you think yeah right, what I really need is a jetpack [sarcastic] because a jet pack allows you to do everything that you are doing now PLUS you'd have a jet pack, you'd be a person with a jet pack [...] The able-bodied think of AT as a form of magic, but we all understand that it is a hardware improvisation and collaboration between the technology and the client [...] Unrealistic goals are seen as the only virtuous and righteous goals [...] It is hard to get them out of the magic notion[...] these two competing mythologies are inhibiting us [...] It is easier to get a grant for a jet pack than it is for a device that gets peas off the plate.

Having unrealistic expectations of the power of technology can have damaging consequences for people with disabilities. One high-profile example of this in the UK is the case of a policeman, called Phillip Olds, who in the 1980s was shot in the line of duty. His injuries left him paralysed. Phillip did not embrace the technology that was available to him at the time, a manual wheelchair. He wanted to be able to walk upright. A national newspaper became aware of his quest and sponsored him to travel to the United States to try out a new wearable computer-controlled device that stimulated the leg muscles (Petrofsky & Phillips, 1983). A national TV station filmed Phillip during and after these trials and broadcast several high-profile documentaries. Unfortunately, the walking aid did not do what Phillip wanted it to do. This was partly because the aid was just an experimental prototype, and partly because Phillip had what could be considered unrealistic expectations about the extent to which the walking aid would render his disability invisible. Sadly, Phillip took his own life. In reflecting on what might be learnt from his experience, Ken Davis, a disabled activist, argued that the able-bodied media were complicit in encouraging Phillip to believe that the walking aid would cure his disability (Davis, 1986). His girlfriend, Vanessa, shared how Phillip did not like the fact that the walking aid marked him out as different.

> When we came back to England, we had already realised that things weren't quite what we had expected. When you talk about research projects, which the walking system was, we thought perhaps that it was going to be a bit further down the road than what it actually was and that the walking with the electronics wasn't going to be quite so crude. What I'd hoped for, having seen the brace, was that he would use it like putting on a pair of trousers. He would put his brace on in the morning and be able to use it when he went to work and he would be back up with 'upright man'. It just didn't work out that way. It was something that he had to put on. Something that was noticeable, made him different from everybody else, as being disabled. It could be that the expectations were too high and had fallen so short; that he didn't want to use it. It wasn't what he was seeking.[4]

The views and experiences of people with disabilities such as John Hockenberry and Phillip Olds are an important reminder to current and prospective researchers in the disability and technology field of the need to be supremely cognisant of how we position and communicate the aims of our research as well as the ethics of what we promise to stakeholders about what can be achieved and when this might be achieved. With this in mind, the underpinning philosophy that runs throughout this book is that technologies have an important role in the lives of people with disabilities, but no matter how 'high-tech' and well-designed these technologies are, they cannot, on their own, transform the lives of people with disabilities.

For over 50 years technologies have been lauded as innovations that would dramatically improve the lives of disabled people. Yet, despite the many new technologies that researchers and developers have produced, people with disabilities are still significantly disadvantaged in society, compared to people without disabilities. Technology has not been the instant agent for inclusion and social justice that many claimed or hoped it would be. Although this has not stopped national and international agencies from investing in future research and development, it should perhaps cause them to evaluate what kinds of research they want to fund in the future. This edited book seeks to address this question. By reviewing research and development literature and presenting case studies of current and past research projects, this book seeks to identify what the particular challengers in the field are at the moment and how they might be addressed in order to map out an agenda for research in the field of disability and technology for the next ten years.

Notes

1. World Health Organization (2023). Assistive Technology. https://www.who.int/news-room/fact-sheets/detail/assistive-technology#:~:text=Assistive%20products%20maintain%20or%20improve,all%20examples%20of%20assistive%20products.
2. World Health Organization (2016). Priority Assistive Products List. https://www.who.int/publications/i/item/priority-assistive-products-list.
3. The speech that John Hockenberry gave was at the 2001 CSUN conference. At the time, it was recorded and placed on this website: http://www.abletv.net/csun2001events.asp. Sadly, the website no longer exists. However, John did publish an autobiography in 1996 called *Moving Violations: War Zones, Wheelchairs, and Declarations of Independence* which covers similar themes.
4. Vanessa Perkins was interviewed for a BBC documentary which aired in the UK in 1995 called *Disabled Lives: Altered States*. See: http://bufvc.ac.uk/dvdfind/index.php/title/5713

References

Davis, K. (1986). Pressed to Death. *Coalition*, December 1986 ,4–5. Greater Manchester Coalition of Disabled People.

Petrofsky, J.S., & Phillips, C.A. (1983). Computer controlled walking in the paralyzed individual. *Journal of Neurological and Orthopaedic Surgery*, 4(2), 153–164.

Seale, J. (2020). Were we right? A re-evaluation of the perceived potential of technology to transform the educational opportunities and outcomes of learners with special educational needs. *History of Education*, 49(2), 247–264.

Seale, J. (2019). Wilderness and resistance: Illuminating the digital inequalities experienced by adults with learning disabilities between 1970 and 1999. *Disability & Society*, 34(9–10), 1481–1503.

Notes

References

1. Constructions of disability and technology and the shaping of future research

Jane Seale

Introduction

The disability and technology community is large and comprises many disciplines and professions. Each stakeholder group has different definitions and constructions of disability and technology and uses different language to describe and categorise them. This can place barriers in the way of collaborative research endeavours. In this chapter I will outline the variations in definitions and constructions of disability and technology and consider the implications for developing a future research agenda. I will also signpost how other chapters in this edited book contribute to or illuminate the debates in the field regarding a lack of shared language and understanding in relation to disability and technology.

Definitions and constructions of disability

The development, use and evaluation of technologies for and by people with disabilities is highly influenced by the models of disability that different stakeholders use to underpin their research, practice or policy as well as the assumptions they hold about people with disabilities as a whole, and the language they use to label them.

Paradigm Shifts in Models of Disability

For many, disability is understood through the models that are operated in educational, health and social welfare settings. Individualistic models of disability are built on the assumption that the problems and difficulties that people with disabilities experience are a direct result of their individual physical, sensory or intellectual impairments. One key example of this kind of model is the medical model, which views disability in terms of disease processes, abnormality and personal tragedy. With the medical model, disability need arises directly from impairment and the major task of the professional is to adjust the individual to the particular disabling condition.

Another example is the charity model of disability which emphasises the personal tragedy of disability. This model is criticised for portraying people with disabilities as helpless, sad and in need of care and protection. Such portrayals are argued to perpetuate damaging stereotypes and misconceptions. This has prompted some charities to move towards using more positive images to portray (and thus define) disability in their fund-raising campaigns and promotional work.

Administrative models of disability usually relate to specific areas of life such as education or employment and are used to assess whether or not people are eligible for certain benefits or accommodations (such as provision of assistive technologies). The associated definitions of disability are written into legislation with legal implications and are viewed by many to be rigid and dichotomous. The definitions almost always relate to people's impairments rather than their physical or social environments. Health and welfare professions are often required to work within the framework of administrative definitions, but critics of this model argue that people with disabilities rarely fit into the neat boxes that administrators provide.

The social model of disability, put forward by disability activists in the United Kingdom, was a move against viewing people with disabilities as dependent and in need of care (Oliver, 1990). Disability was viewed as stemming from failure of the social and physical environment to take account of people with disabilities' needs. The problems of people with disabilities were therefore not seen as within the individual person, but within society. According to the social model, it is not the individual with a disability that needs to be changed, but society. Impairment therefore is an individual limitation, while a disability is a socially imposed restriction. Not being able to walk is an impairment, but lack of mobility is a disability (a socially created situation).

The influence of the social and medical models of disability can also be seen in the development of classification systems that attempt to distinguish between impairment and disability. One example is the International Classification of Impairment, Disability and Handicap (ICDH), first developed by the World Health Organization in 1980. This classification initially had a very medical focus, where handicap and disability were seen as a problem of the person and caused by disease or trauma. Impairments were defined as a consequence of disease or disorder; disability was defined as a consequence of impairments and handicap was defined as a consequence of disabilities.

Influenced by the social model, the World Health Organization began to re-develop its classification in the late 1990s. This new classification facilitated a merger between the medical and social model and attempted to include environmental factors. Disability was now seen as an interaction between health conditions and contextual factors where both factors influence the activities that a disabled person can perform or participate in.

Disability was therefore understood as the extent to which performance of activities is limited. Activity was defined as everything that a person does. Participation was defined as the interaction of impairments, disabilities and contextual factors and comprises all aspects of human life. Contextual factors were defined as the complete background to a person's life and living, including external environmental factors and internal personal factors. In 2011, the World Health Organization adopted a new classification, the International Classification of Functioning, Disability and Health (ICF), which reaffirmed the social determinants of disability and stated that disability is a function of one's interaction with individual, institutional and social environments (WHO, 2011). In the proceeding years the World Health Organization has maintained its commitment to this biopsychosocial model of disability which conceptualises a person's level of functioning as a dynamic interaction between her or his health conditions, environmental factors and personal factors (WHO & UNICEF, 2022). The ICF therefore defines 'impairments' as problems in body function or structure such as a significant deviation or loss. 'Activity limitations' are defined as difficulties an individual may have in executing a task or action, and 'participation restrictions' are defined as problems an individual may experience in involvement in life situations. The ICF uses 'functioning' when referring to all body functions, activities and participation, and uses 'disability' as an umbrella term for impairments, activity limitations and participation restrictions.

The shift towards recognising interactions between individual, environmental and social factors is reflected in the United Nations (UN) Convention on the Rights of Persons with Disabilities (UN, 2006) which states that "persons with disabilities include those who have long-term physical, mental, intellectual or sensory impairments which in interaction with various barriers may hinder their full and effective participation in society on an equal basis with others". We can also see the influence of this shift on disability and technology research. For example, in tracing the history of the 'Universal Design of ICT',

Begnum (2020) credits the shift in disability perspective from a medical model to a psychosocial and situated model as influencing the move away from specialised adaptations and add-on assistive technologies towards universal solutions. Newbutt and Bradley (2022) argue that using participatory design methods that involve autistic children and young people in research into the applications of immersive virtual reality represents a 'paradigm shift' away from medical-based models of disability because they value the voice and opinions of the technology user rather than medical or rehabilitation professionals. Tsatsou (2021) argues that the barriers to digital inclusion experienced by people with disabilities are determined by complex biopsychosocial factors and therefore recommends that digital inclusion researchers adopt the biopsychosocial model of disability, in order to generate useful insights.

The shift in disability paradigms or models is not universal across the Assistive Technology (AT) field, however. For example, writing in the context of Artificial Intelligence (AI) development, Newman-Griffis et al. (2023) argue that there are three interlocking mechanisms that support ableism in AI development, one of which is the prevalence of a medicalised conception of disability:

> Disabled people are neither assumed to be nor hired to work as creators and designers of AI technologies, excluding them from having agency in the development and evaluation of AI technologies with direct impact on their lives. [...] This is intertwined with the curative goals that often drive conceptualisation and implementation of health-related AI technologies (i.e., that they will be used to help cure or fix the "harm" of disability), which are often based on normative assumptions of disability as deviation from a desired social norm. Moreover, disability is often treated as a monolith (e.g., seeking input from arbitrary "disabled" users, regardless of individual experience), which does not represent the multidimensionality of collective experience or practice. (p. 5)

Newman-Griffis et al. (2023) challenge the AI community to develop processes that do not require people with disabilities to conform to a disabled world. Such a challenge should probably also apply to any new technologies that we develop as part of our research agenda for the next ten years.

Contesting Disability Assumptions and Language

Although there has been a shift from classifying individual deficits to acknowledging the social, political and cultural barriers that serve to marginalise people with disabilities, disability remains a contested concept. For example, writing in the context of automated decision-making and digital inclusion, Goggin and Soldatić (2022) contest the assumption that people with disabilities are a homogenous population. They argue that while there might be commonalities in relation to digital exclusion and inequalities that people with disabilities experience, there will also be differences that are influenced by a "complex set of embodied, affective, social, political, and cultural identities, experiences and subjectivities" (p. 387).

Another area of contestation is the use of language. Language reflects the cultural assumptions and thinking of the society around us. Language is therefore never purely descriptive; it shapes how we see each other, the value we place on different identities, and sometimes how we behave. This is why proponents of the social model of disability rejected terms such as 'handicapped', 'retarded' or 'wheelchair-bound' because they reflected a negative or medical view of disability. Arguing for more positive language, the social model proposed terms such as 'disabled person' (not 'handicapped'), 'person with learning disabilities' (not 'retarded') and 'wheelchair user' (not 'wheelchair-bound').

More recently, there has been debate regarding whether it is appropriate to use identity-first language or person-first language. Identity-first language prioritises a disability label as a statement of identity (for example, 'autistic person' as opposed to 'person with autism'). Identity-first language signifies identification with a collective cultural identity. Sometimes, as in the case of autism or deafness, it is an identity that people are incredibly proud of. In addition, capitalisation (e.g. d/Deaf person) is a political statement that is used to emphasise and signify the shared, disabling experience that people with impairments face in society. Person-first language (e.g. 'person with a learning disability') places the term 'person' before the disability diagnosis. This language is typically employed as a reaction against dehumanising labels such as 'cripple' or 'retard' and challenges the world to see the person first and the disability second.

It is also important to be aware that there are international differences in the use of disability-related terms. For example, in the UK the term 'learning disability' is preferred to the term 'intellectual impairment' or 'intellectual disability' which is used in other countries. Sometimes in the field the term 'learning disability' includes autism, sometimes it does not. Sometimes the term 'cognitive impairment' is used as an all-encompassing term that includes people with learning disabilities, people with dementia and people with traumatic brain injury. Therefore, it is important when researching in this field to make absolutely clear which populations or groups are being referred to and how these might relate to other relevant groups.

Definitions and constructions of technology

In the disability and technology community there are disagreements and tensions regarding the extent to which designers should be focused on designing specialist or mainstream technologies and the potential risks of being overly enthusiastic about the potential of technologies to transform the lives of people with disabilities. Alongside this, there are international variations in how technologies are labelled or categorised.

Debates Regarding the Need for both Specialist and Mainstream Technologies

Prior to the emergence of Universal Design (UD) and similar design approaches, technologies used to be divided into two categories: mainstream and specialist; where mainstream technologies were those that were not designed with the needs of people with disabilities in mind. Many of these would be labelled as either Information and Communication Technologies (ICT) or Information Technologies (IT). Specialist technologies were often labelled as 'assistive technologies' and were specifically designed with the needs of specific disability groups in mind (e.g. alternative and augmentative communication aids). Specialist or assistive technologies typically looked very different and there is a large body of literature reporting how people with disabilities found these technologies stigmatising and therefore were reluctant to use them (see for example Roulstone, 2016).

Over time, with improved design and the emergence of UD principles (Center for Universal Design, 1997) many (although not all) mainstream technologies have become more accessible. Alongside this, the definition of what constitutes assistive technology has broadened considerably to include any product or service that can increase, maintain or improve a person's functional capabilities and improve their quality of life. For example, the WHO and UNICEF (2022) define AT as:

> an umbrella term for assistive products and their related systems and services. Assistive technology enables and promotes the inclusion, participation and engagement of persons with disabilities, ageing populations and people living with chronic conditions in the family, community and all areas of society, including the political, economic and social spheres. Assistive products can enhance performance in all key functional domains such as cognition, communication, hearing, mobility, self-care and vision. (p. xi)

This has led some to argue that there is no longer a need for designers to develop specialist technologies. Others argue that although adopting UD principles might reduce the need for specialist technologies, it will never totally eliminate the need. Some people with disabilities will have access needs that simply cannot be met by mainstream technologies.

Tensions between Techno-centric and Techno-sceptic Constructions of Technology

In the research and practice literature there is a long history of techno-centric enthusiasm regarding the potential of technology to improve the lives of people with disabilities. Technologies and technology designs have persistently been described as innovatory with the potential to have a positive influence on the lives of people with disabilities. For example, in the 1980s microcomputer technology was heralded as having huge potential to revolutionise learning, particularly for children with physical, sensory and cognitive impairments. For example, Cain (1984) considered that microcomputer technology represented the most "revolutionary innovation yet developed in the field of education" (p. 239). Goldman et al. (1987) argued that microcomputer technology was the latest in a series of "instructional innovations to be touted as the answer to educational problems" (p. 331). While references to revolutionary trans-formation have been toned down, the discourse of innovation still exists in current research and practice literature. For example, writing in the context of developing mobility solutions, Banes et al. (2020) propose that: "Recent innovations in both assistive and accessible technologies, such as natural interfaces, wearable technologies and artificial intelligence suggest new ways in which navigation, orientation and wayfinding can be made accessible for people with a variety of needs, including those with cognitive, sensory, physical impairments and the elderly" (p. 277).

Kamalakannan et al. (2023) describe their proposed digital therapeutic platform for people with stroke-related disabilities as an innovation. In a self-confessed sceptical tone, Goggin and Soldatić (2022) suggest that disability is often given as a warrant for the introduction of new technology, which can lead to disability becoming a "a major zone for technology innovation, development, application, design and so on" (p. 385). This is suggestive perhaps of the phe-nomenon of 'technology going in search of a problem', where designers and others have decided they want to develop a particular technology and latch onto disability as the justification for doing so, rather than seeking to under-stand the difficulties people with disabilities face and developing technologies to address specific needs or desires.

The discourse of innovation has been accompanied in the literature by a nar-rative that positions technology as a prosthetic or a panacea. Many in the disability and technology community are critical of this narrative and have proposed alternative narratives such as: technology is a tool; or technology is a double-edged sword.

Technology as a prosthetic or panacea

Early on in the history of designing new technologies for people with disabilities, practitioners and researchers heralded technology as providing an emancipatory breakthrough for people with disabilities. One example is the field of education:

> This new technology can emancipate the handicapped and help to open up the horizons of many children whose communication and interaction with the outside world were previously very limited. (Southgate, 1985, p. 150)

> For pupils with significant physical and sensory impairments, IT can provide physical access to the curriculum. This is technology at its most dramatic, liberating the pupil from the physical barriers to learning [...] For these pupils, the technology provides independent access to a world of communication and learning that has been closed until now. It is no wonder then that we consider IT in the context of physical access as a lifeline. (Day, 1995, p. 4)

This narrative led to a tendency to position technology as something that can solve the problem of impairment, by either acting as a prosthetic and compensating for a person's disability or acting as a panacea, something that can fix or cure a person's disability. One consequence of this is that stakeholders over-focused on the technological wizardry of the new products being developed and ignored the perceptions and experiences of people with disabilities themselves as well as the personal and social factors that can influence the success or failure of technology use. Many people with disabilities warned that viewing technology as miraculous was discriminatory because it emphasised "the otherness accompanying disability" (Fisher, 1993, p. 17). Smith (1989), a technology user with physical disabilities, stated:

> Technology is always going to be crucial importance to me, but it isn't everything. In my view technology, used with care and the right kind of support, can help towards independence but over-emphasis on it can smother an individual's resources and only lead in the end to further limitations. (p. 190)

Grijseels et al. (2021) argue that the positioning of technology as capable of transformational fixes persists in current policy discourses: "Following conventional dichotomies, policy actors generally consider technologies to either provide a prosthetic fix to 'able' people with disabilities or become instruments for social transformation" (p. 1).

Disability and technology scholars have commented on how viewing technology as a prosthesis or panacea reflects a medical or rehabilitation view of disability which overamplifies the benefits of technology and seeks to eradicate or deny the existence of disability. For example, Roulstone (2016) writes that such views "misread the benefits of technology and offer misplaced hope as to the potential of technology" (p. 1), while Shildrick (2002) problematises the assumption that people with disabilities would want to use technologies in order to escape from their disabled bodies. In an examination of how disability has an intertwined history with the history of computing, Wu (2021) offers an example from the late 1980s to illustrate their argument that disability was seen as a problem to fix:

> Most of these cybernetic prostheses were designed against, rather than with, disability. Wiener's "hearing glove," for instance, was based on his belief that "deaf-mutes" produced speech with "a grotesque and harsh intonation," which was a "highly inefficient form" of communication. The "hearing glove" was thus more about making d/Deaf people speak legibly to hearing people than facilitating mutual communication. Projects like this showcased the prowess of cybernetic innovation by making disabled body-minds "normal". (p. 68)

Despite their criticisms of extreme techno-centric constructions, most disability and technology scholars do not dismiss the potential of technology, rather they counsel for caution and the need for more research in order to develop a greater understanding of the relationship between people with disabilities and their technologies. For example, Swartz and Marchetti-Mercer (2019) argue:

> Disability scholars need to study what technology can and cannot do, and we also need to be aware of ways in which the dazzling success of technology can have unintended consequences. These consequences are varied, but two worth mentioning here are the denial of the body and its needs, and the re-inscribing of the non-normative body as a problem which technology can, and should, cure or circumvent. (p. 417)

Technology as a tool

In the 1980s and 1990s, key influential figures in the special education field in the UK were concerned that overly techno-centric constructions of technology would lead to unrealistic expectations of what technology could achieve for learners with a disability and urged teachers and parents not to view technology as a panacea. Heddell (1985) wrote that "[m]icrocomputers can sometimes help; they cannot work miracles" (p. 2). Hawkridge and Vincent (1992) wrote that while computers "can help learners to overcome their difficulties. They cannot work magic. They are not necessarily the best solution" (p. 21). With this narrative came the introduction of the metaphor of microtechnology as a tool; something that could extend the ability of a person with a disability to accomplish a particular task:

> We have to decide if new technology is a miracle cure-all or if it is just the flavour of the month and can be safely ignored […] reality lies at neither of these extremes, but […] computers can in the right circumstances, be very powerful tools in helping children with learning difficulties. (Hope, 1987, p. 13)

In 2019, I interviewed teachers, advisors and researchers who had worked in special education since the 1970s about the role of technology, then and now (Seale, 2019). I noticed a more nuanced use of the term 'tool' when referring to technology. Many participants were keen not to overplay the potential of technology and seemed to want not to overstate its power by referring to it as *'just* a tool'.

The use of the term 'tool' as a metaphor to describe technology persists today across the whole AT field. For example Griffin et al. (2020) refer to a Virtual Reality program for pain intervention as a tool to "facilitate therapeutic gains in chronic pain rehabilitation in a manner that is highly reinforcing and fun" (p. 1). Winberg et al. (2021) conducted focus groups with 16 older people with a range of neurological disabilities (e.g. stroke, multiple sclerosis or Parkinson's disease) about how they felt about using mobile technology apps to facilitate self-management tasks (e.g. monitor and manage symptoms). They also refer to these apps as tools, although it is interesting that the participants did not appear to do so. Many website developers and accessibility researchers talk about tools that can help to make websites more accessible (see for example Kumar et al., 2021).

Technology as a double-edged sword

In the disability and technology literature there is a persistent tension regarding the fact that technologies can have both a positive and a negative impact on people with disabilities. For example Lupton and Seymour (2000) interviewed 15 people with physical disabilities living in Adelaide, Australia, about the contribution of technology to their lives. The participants identified both positive and negative aspects of technology. On the one hand many technologies were highly beneficial, allowing them to "transcend some aspects of their disabilities" (p. 1851). On the other hand they could also have a negative impact, by serving to "mark out people with disabilities as 'different' or 'lacking', acting as a barrier to the achievement and presentation of their preferred body/self" (p. 1851). Such experiences led Goggin (2018) to argue that we need to navigate the tensions between being overly fixated on the potential benefits of technology and ignoring the role those digital technologies play in inequalities. Arguments like these suggest that we need therefore to seek to understand technology as both an enabler and disabler, a double-edged sword. Writing in the context of accessibility, Katseva (2004) claimed that:

> Technology is a double-edged blade: it can empower, or it can disable. Technology empowers when it levels the playing field by rendering disabilities irrelevant in a given context. In this case, it fosters equality. However, technology disables when it is developed without considering accessibility because it marginalizes segments of the population.

Bryen et al. (2007) apply the metaphor to the use of technologies by people with intellectual disabilities:

> Technology acts as a double-edged sword for people with intellectual disabilities. On the one hand, it incorporates many characteristics that are inherent barriers to such people (e.g., complexity, high cost, requirements for literacy, and demands for increased speed of decision-making). At the same time, technology contains the as-yet-unrealized potential to overcome many of these same barriers. (p. 6)

Variations in Technology Terms and Labels

It is important to acknowledge that internationally there are variations in the terms and labels applied to technology. For example, in Germany and the United States the term 'rehabilitative technology' is used to refer to technologies that help people recover or improve function after injury or illness. Examples include robotics (e.g. Jyräkoski et al., 2021) and virtual reality (e.g. Griffin et al., 2020). In Sweden, the term 'welfare technology' is commonly used. Although there is no official definition of welfare technology, Borg et al. (2023) indicate that it is commonly understood to mean any technology that maintains or increases the safety, activity, participation or independence of people with disabilities. Gauci (2021) chooses to use the term 'enabling technology' and defines this as including both assistive technology and mainstream technology. Their justification for this is because "the distinction between mainstream and AT has greatly blurred since we are living in an age of integrated technology. It is very difficult to separate the two" (p. 489).

Sometimes in research, technology is categorised in different ways depending on how people with disabilities use them. For example, Egard and Hansson (2021) observed and interviewed adults with various disabilities in Sweden about their use of different digital technologies. Their analysis suggested that technologies could be categorised as either 'spontaneous' or 'imperative'. Spontaneous technologies were those that participants had voluntarily introduced into their lives for work or pleasure, and which typically made their lives easier. Examples included smartphones and computers. Imperative technologies were those that participants were forced to use by service providers, and which did not necessarily make their lives easier. Examples included online shopping and booking services. Pedersen et al. (2019) use the phrase 'assistive activity technology' (AAT) which they defined as any technology that is designed specifically to help individuals with impairments participate in physical activities. These include outdoor activities, exercise, sports, play and physical education. Some examples of AAT are adjusted bikes, alpine equipment, wheelchairs modified for playing tennis or dancing, and hockey sleds.

Implications for scoping a future research agenda

In outlining the variations in definitions and constructions of disability and technology I have highlighted how disability and technology are not neutral concepts. In the disability and technology community they provoke a range of responses. Therefore, in order for us to produce an agenda for future research that is going to be meaningful, relevant and accepted by this community it is important to demonstrate an awareness of the tensions and sensitivities. Sometimes this might mean adopting new practices, sometimes it might mean avoiding particular practices and sometimes it might mean taking the time to justify certain practices or positions.

Our awareness of the paradigm shifts in models of disability may lead us to develop a particular focus on reducing environmental and societal barriers to accessing and using technologies. In seeking to be careful of the assumptions we make about the homogeneity of people with disabilities as a group it may be important not to assume that people with the same disability label have the same technology needs or experience or face similar inequalities to people with different disability labels.

If we believe that there is a need for a specialist piece of technology to be developed in the future, that is likely to meet the access needs of a relatively small group of people with disabilities, we may need to develop design practices that ensure the extensive involvement of people from the target community so that the resulting technology is not considered 'stigmatising'.

We also need to be aware that people with disabilities are likely to use a wide range of technologies in their daily lives; some mainstream, some more specialist, some spontaneous, some imperative. Part of what we might need to research and understand is how people with disabilities cope with an ecology of interconnected technologies (Kobbelgaard et al., 2020). For example, Buchholz et al. (2020) report that some people with 'communicative and cognitive disabilities' find it difficult to switch between their specialist Alternative or Augmentative Communication software and the more mainstream software that they also use, because this requires skills that not all users or support persons have.

We also need to be careful to think about the consequences of being overly techno-centric about the potential impact or value of technologies in the lives of people with disabilities and ignore the social factors that shape their use of technologies. A powerful example of this is provided by research into the reactions of d/Deaf people to cochlear implants. In the d/d/Deaf community there are disagreements over whether d/Deaf people should embrace cochlear implants, with some arguing strongly that they are proud of their d/Deaf identity and do not wish to seek to deny that identity by using the implants (Ahlin & Hiddinga, 2023; Chang & Tucker, 2022; Salehomoum, 2020; Mauldin, 2019). For example, Salehomoum (2020) interviewed 11 d/Deaf adults in the US about why they had decided to stop using their cochlear implant. Results indicated that several factors played a role in their abandonment of the implants, but one of the most prominent factors was challenges in negotiating a d/d/Deaf identity. The d/Deaf participants talked about their dislike of being pushed to use speech as opposed to sign language and feeling a sense of 'in-betweenness', neither belonging to the d/Deaf community or the hearing community. Most had made the decision to abandon their impact during early to late adolescence, a time when many of us are grappling with our identity and how we want to see ourselves in the future. Interestingly, eight of the interviewees described their implant as a device or tool. Interview responses also consistently indicated that an implant is not a fix.

Finally, the variations and disagreements over the language used to refer to disability and technology presents a major challenge to the field of disability and technology. A large number of stakeholders operate in this field and often they are required to collaborate in AT research and development. If these stakeholders do not have a shared language that is widely understood and accepted, then the likelihood of misunderstandings and disagreements is high, putting at risk the completion of research projects that could potentially move the field forward.

Conclusion and preview

In this chapter I have highlighted how definitions and constructions of disability and technology vary in the field and argued that this has important implications for the development of a future research agenda. In this book, prominent researchers in the field will draw on their personal research experiences and projects. In doing so, they will provide further context and evidence for this argument as well as illuminate some of the tensions and sensitivities that I have outlined in this chapter.

The paradigmatic shifts in how disability is constructed have implications for how we involve people with disabilities in the design of technologies. In Chapter 3, Alan Foley describes and evaluates the Participatory Action Research approach that was implemented in a design project involving users with intellectual disabilities. He discusses how the culture of 'ableism' within the institution where the project took place presented particular barriers or challenges. In Chapter 9, I report on the results of a critical review of studies that have involved people with disabilities in the design of new technologies. Both chapters prompt us to consider how to involve people with disabilities in the design of technologies so that we focus less on their perceived deficits and more on the skills and expertise that they bring to the design project.

Some of the chapter authors will use language or terms that may be unfamiliar to us but are meaningful in the context in which they are working. For example, in Chapter 6, Robert McLaren, Shamima Akhtar and Clive Gilbert coin the term 'ATech' to refer to accessible and assistive technology. In Chapter 8, Rohan Slaughter, Annalu Waller and Tom Griffiths use the term 'Educational Assistive Technology'. However, in talking about the role of technology in the lives of people with disabilities, none of the chapter authors use language that might suggest they are positioning technology as a panacea or miracle cure. Implicit in much of what they say is the acceptance that without good designs, good support practices and inclusive environments people with disabilities will not be able to benefit from accessing and using technologies.

A number of the chapters address the debates that exist regarding the need for both specialist and mainstream technologies. In Chapter 4, Paul Whittington and Huseyin Dogan describe the designs they have produced in response to the challenges that people with disabilities experience authenticating themselves or communicating their accessibility requirements through traditional methods, such as Personal Identification Number (PIN) codes or textual passwords. The design of one of their apps, EduAbility, has been influenced by the belief that there is not a single solution to fit multiple needs. In Chapter 7, Dave Edyburn critically analyses the assistive technology service delivery system in order to identify novel approaches to automating assistive technology data collection and analysis. To underpin this critique he considers the drivers for change in the AT field and notes the unresolved tensions between UD and AT. In Chapter 8, Rohan Slaughter, Annalu Waller and Tom Griffiths discuss what they consider to be the limits of the UD approach and also what 'mainstreaming' of AT means in current times.

In reading this and the other contributing chapters, it is my hope that readers will carefully examine the language they use, the assumptions that they have about the power of technology and the agency of people with disabilities and how their personal constructions of disability and technology might influence the research questions that they seek to answer and the R&D methods they implement. If disability and technology are not neutral, neither are we as researchers and developers.

References

Ahlin, T., & Hiddinga, A. (2023). Technological socialities: The impact of information and communication technologies on belonging among deaf and hard-of-hearing people. *Sociology Compass*, e13068. https://doi.org/10.1111/soc4.13068

Banes, D., Magni, R., & Brinkmann, F. (2020). Implementation and Innovation in the Area of Independent Mobility Through Digital Technologies. In Miesenberger, K., Manduchi, R., Covarrubias Rodriguez, M., & Peňáz, P. (Eds.), *Computers Helping People with Special Needs. ICCHP 2020. Lecture Notes in Computer Science, vol 12377* (pp. 199–206). Springer. https://doi.org/10.1007/978-3-030-58805-2_33

Begnum, M.E.N. (2020). Universal Design of ICT: A Historical Journey from Specialized Adaptations Towards Designing for Diversity. In Antona, M., & Stephanidis, C. (Eds.), *Universal Access in Human-Computer Interaction. Design Approaches and Supporting Technologies. HCII 2020. Lecture Notes in Computer Science, vol 12188* (pp. 3–18). Springer. https://doi.org/10.1007/978-3-030-49282-3_1

Borg, J., Gustafsson, C., Stridsberg, S.L., & Zander, V. (2023). Implementation of welfare technology: A state-of-the-art review of knowledge gaps and research needs. *Disability and Rehabilitation: Assistive Technology*, 18(2), 227–239. DOI:10.1080/17483107.2022.2120104

Bryen, D.N., Carey, A., & Friedman, M. (2007). Cell phone use by adults with intellectual disabilities. *Intellectual and Developmental Disabilities*, 45(1), 1–9. DOI:10.1352/1934-9556(2007)45[1:CPUBAW]2.0.CO;2

Buchholz, M., Holmgren, K., & Ferm, U. (2020). Remote communication for people with disabilities: Support persons' views on benefits, challenges, and suggestions for technology development. *Technology & Disability*, 32(2), 69–80. DOI:10.3233/TAD-190254

Cain, E.J. (1984). The challenge of technology: Educating the exceptional child for the world of tomorrow. *Teaching Exceptional Children, 16*(4), 239–241.

Center for Universal Design (1997). *Principles of Universal Design.* https://design.ncsu.edu/research/center-for-universal-design/

Chang, P.F., & Tucker, R.V. (2022). Assistive communication technologies and stigma: How perceived visibility of cochlear implants affects self-stigma and social interaction anxiety. *Proceedings of the ACM on Human-Computer Interaction, 6*(CSCW1), 1–16. https://doi.org/10.1145/3512924

Day, J. (1995). *Access Technology: Making the Right Choice.* NCET.

Egard, H., & Hansson, K. (2021). The digital society comes sneaking in. An emerging field and its disabling barriers. *Disability & Society, 38*(5), 761–775. DOI:10.1080/09687599.2021.1960275

Fisher, P. (1993). Enabling the disabled. *The Guardian,* 24 June, p. 17.

Gauci, V. (2021). Dis/ability-producing technology assemblages and networks at the workplace: A new materialist analysis. *Disability & Society, 36*(3), 488–507. DOI:10.1080/09687599.2020.1758038

Goggin, G., & Soldatić, K. (2022). Automated decision-making, digital inclusion and intersectional disabilities. *New Media & Society, 24*(2), 384–400.

Goggin, G. (2018). Disability & Digital Inequalities: Rethinking Digital Divides with Disability Theory. In Ragnedda, M., & Muschert, G.W. (Eds.), *Theorizing Digital Divides* (pp. 63–74). Routledge.

Goldman, S.R., Semmel., D.S., Cosden, M.A., Gerber, M.M., & Semmel, M.I. (1987). Special education administrator's policies and practices on microcomputer acquisition, allocation and access for mildly handicapped children. *Exceptional Children, 53*(4), 330–339.

Griffin, A., Wilson, L., Feinstein A.B., Bortz, A., Heirich, M.S., Gilkerson, R., Wagner, J.F.M., Menendez, M., Caruso, T.J., Rodriguez, S., Naidu, S., Golianu, B., & Simons, L.E. (2020). Virtual reality in pain rehabilitation for youth with chronic pain: Pilot feasibility study. *JMIR Rehabilitation and Assistive Technologies, 7*(2): e22620. https://rehab.jmir.org/2020/2/e22620/

Grijseels, M., Zuiderent-Jerak, T., & Regeer, B.J. (2021). Technologies for inclusive employment: Beyond the prosthetic fix–social transformation axis. *Disability & Society,* DOI:10.1080/09687599.2021.1997720

Hawkridge, D., & Vincent, T. (1992). *Learning Difficulties and Computers: Access to the Curriculum.* Jessica Kingsley.

Heddell, F. (1985). *With a little help from the chip.* BBC.

Hope, M.H. (1987). *Micros for Children with Special Needs.* Souvenir Press.

Jyräkoski, T., Merilampa, S., Puustinen, J., & Kärki, A. (2021). Over-ground robotic lower limb exoskeleton in neurological gait rehabilitation: User experiences and effects on walking ability. *Technology & Disability, 33*(1), 53–63. DOI:10.3233/TAD-200284

Kamalakannan, S., Karunakaran, V., Balaji, A., Vijaykaran, A.S., Ramachandran, S., & Nagarajan R. (2023). Evaluation of the feasibility and acceptability of ReWin—A digital therapeutic rehabilitation innovation for people with stroke-related disabilities in India. *Frontiers in Neurology,* 13, 936787. DOI:10.3389/fneur.2022.936787

Katseva, A. (2004). The case for pervasive accessibility. Paper presented at the Center on Disabilities: Technology and Persons with Disabilities Conference 2004.

Kobbelgaard, F.V., Bødker, S., & Kanstrup, A.M. (2020). Designing a game to explore human artefact ecologies for assistive robotics: Basing design games on an activity theoretical framework. In *NordiCHI '20: Proceedings of the 11th Nordic Conference* on *Human-Computer Interaction: Shaping Experiences, Shaping Society* (pp. 1–10). Association for Computing Machinery. https://doi.org/10.1145/3419249.3420181

Kumar, S., Shree, D.V.J., & Biswas, P. (2021). Comparing ten WCAG tools for accessibility evaluation of websites. *Technology & Disability, 33*(3), 163–185. DOI:10.3233/TAD-210329

Lupton, D., & Seymour, W. (2000). Technology, selfhood and physical disability. *Social Science & Medicine, 50*(12), 1851–1862. https://doi.org/10.1016/S0277-9536(99)00422-0

Mauldin, L. (2019). Don't look at it as a miracle cure: Contested notions of success and failure in family narratives of pediatric cochlear implantation. *Social Science & Medicine, 228,* 117–125. https://doi.org/10.1016/j.socscimed.2019.03.021

Newbutt, N., & Bradley, R. (2022). Using immersive virtual reality with autistic pupils: Moving towards greater inclusion and co-participation through ethical practices. *Journal of Enabling Technologies, 16*(2), 124–140. https://doi.org/10.1108/JET-01-2022-0010

Newman-Griffis, D., Rauchberg, J.S., Alharbi, R., Hickman, L., & Hochheiser, H. (2023). Definition drives design: Disability models and mechanisms of bias in AI technologies. *First Monday, 28*(1). https://doi.org/10.5210/fm.v28i1.12903

Oliver, M. (1990). *The politics of disablement.* Basingstoke: MacMillan and St Martins Press.

Pedersen, H., Söderström, S., & Kermit, P.S. (2019). Assistive activity technology as symbolic expressions of the self. *Technology and Disability, 31*(3), 129–140. DOI:10.3233/TAD-190236

Roulstone, A. (2016). *Disability & Technology: An Interdisciplinary and International Approach.* Palgrave Macmillan.

Salehomoum, M. (2020). Cochlear implant nonuse: Insight from deaf adults. *The Journal of Deaf Studies and Deaf Education, 25*(3), 270–282. https://doi.org/10.1093/deafed/enaa002

Seale, J. (2019). Wilderness and resistance: Illuminating the digital inequalities experienced by adults with learning disabilities between 1970 and 1999. *Disability & Society, 34*(9–10), 1481–1503. https://doi.org/10.1080/09687599.2019.1576504

Shildrick, M. (2002). *Embodying the Monster: Encounters with the Vulnerable Self.* Sage Publications.

Smith, A. (1989). An individual experience. In Vincent, A.T. (Ed.), *New Technology, Disability and Special Educational Needs* (pp. 188–191). FEU and The Open University.

Southgate, T. (1985). Microcomputer software: Aids to communication. *British Journal of Special Education, 12*(4), 150. DOI:10.1111/j.1467-8578.1985.tb00007.x

Swartz, L., & Marchetti-Mercer, M. (2019). Migration, technology and care: What happens to the body? *Disability & Society, 34*(3), 407–420. DOI:10.1080/09687599.2018.1519409

Tsatsou, P. (2021). Is digital inclusion fighting disability stigma? Opportunities, barriers, and recommendations. *Disability & Society, 36*(5), 702–729. DOI:10.1080/0968 7599.2020.1749563

United Nations (2006). *Convention on the rights of persons with disabilities and optional protocol.* https:// www .un .org/ development/ desa/ disabilities/ convention -on -the -rights-of-persons-with-disabilities.html

WHO (2001) International Classification of Functioning, Disability and Health.

WHO (World Health Organization) & World Bank (2011). *World report on disability.* https:// www .who .int/ teams/ noncommunicable -diseases/ sensory -functions

-disability-and-rehabilitation/world-report-on-disability#:~:text=World%20Report%20on%20Disability%202011,a%20figure%20of%20around%2010%25.

WHO & UNICEF (2022). *Global report on assistive technology.* https://apps.who.int/iris/handle/10665/354357

Winberg, C., Kylberg, M., Pettersson, C., Harnett, T., Hedvall, P-O., Mattsson, T., & Månsson Lexell, E. (2021). Feeling controlled or being in control? Apps for self-management among older people with neurological disability. *Disability and Rehabilitation: Assistive Technology, 16*(6), 603–608. DOI:10.1080/17483107.2019.1685017

Wu, D. (2021). Cripping the history of computing. *IEEE Annals of the History of Computing, 43*(3), 68–72. DOI:10.1109/MAHC.2021.3101061

2.   Scoping a future research agenda for disability and technology: issues to consider

Jane Seale

Introduction

The purpose of this chapter is to provide an overarching review of the factors that will influence the development of a future research agenda; the kinds of issues or challenges that need to be addressed by future research and how the questions that arise from these issues may need to be answered. Two main drivers for disability and technology research will be outlined and discussed: (1) digital exclusion and digital inequalities and (2) capturing outcomes of assistive technology (AT) use. Two potential areas for future research will be discussed: (1) the design, provision and impact of new technologies and (2) the history of technology design, provision and use. The call for more involvement of people with disabilities in AT research and development will be discussed along with the implications this has for how research is conducted in the future. Finally, the chapter will conclude by highlighting how the rest of the contributing book chapters will relate to or expand on the issues that have been identified through the review.

Global drivers for disability and technology research

Globally, there are two main issues that are driving and influencing research in the disability and technology field: (1) digital exclusion and digital inequalities and (2) capturing outcomes of assistive technology use.

Digital Exclusion and Digital Inequalities

For over 20 years, researchers have reported evidence that there is a difference in how people without disabilities and people with disabilities are engaging with and benefitting from technologies (typically the Internet or Information and Communications Technology (ICT)). There is also evidence to indicate that there are differences between different disability groups. Research has revealed a number of barriers to digital inclusion, many of which are contributing to significant inequalities between the Global North and the Global South. It is widely agreed that addressing the digital marginalisation of people with disabilities requires policy interventions in order to drive broader structural changes in society and across the globe.

Differences in technology access and use between people with and without disabilities

Numerous studies in the United States (US) have found that people with disabilities lag behind those without disabilities in access to computers and the Internet (Kaye, 2000; National Telecommunications and Information Administration, 2002). This lag is persistent over time. Dobransky and Hargittai (2006) used data collected by the Bureau of Labor Statistics and the Census of the United States to examine differences in computer ownership, Internet access and Internet use. They found people with disabilities were less likely to live in households with computers, less likely to use computers and less likely to be online. Dobransky and Hargittai (2016) analysed the US Federal Communication Commission's 2009 National Consumer Broadband Service Capability Survey (NCBSCS) in order to answer the question: is there a divide between people with disabilities and those without disabilities in basic Internet access, holding other sociodemographic factors constant? They reported that significantly fewer people with disabilities use the Internet compared to people without disabilities; among those people with access to the Internet, 67 per cent of people with disabilities reported high-speed, broadband connections, compared with 78 per cent of those without disabilities; even when demographic and socioeconomic variables such as age, income and education are controlled for, those reporting a disability had considerably lower odds of accessing the Internet.

In a follow-up study, Dobransky and Hargittai (2021) compared the data from the 2009 NCBSCS survey with data that they collected in 2020 as part of a study about how people in the US were coping with the covid-19 pandemic. Their particular focus was comparing the Internet skills of respondents with and without disabilities and assessing whether there was a difference and if this difference had decreased over time. They found that in 2009, people with disabilities reported lower skills than people without disabilities, but that in 2020 the difference between the two groups was no longer significant. They suggest that one reason for this reduction is that technology firms have improved the accessibility of their products. However, they also caution that digital skills is just one measure of the digital divide and that digital inequalities still need to be addressed. Scanlan (2022) analysed data from the 2017 Current Population Survey in the US in order to examine whether people with disabilities own computers, connect to the Internet and participate in online activities at the same rates as the general population. They found that people with disabilities are less likely than others to participate in many online activities. Areas where they lag include using the Internet for E-mail, texting/instant messaging, shopping, hiring services, and banking/finance.

Examining data from 2017, the Office for National Statistics (ONS) in the United Kingdom reported that across all age groups, adults with disabilities made up a large proportion of adult Internet non-users. Adults with disabilities comprised 56 per cent of adult Internet non-users which was much higher than the proportion of adults with disabilities in the UK population as a whole, which in 2016 to 2017 was estimated to be 22 per cent (ONS, 2019). Longitudinal research by Helsper and Reisdorf (2017) compared Internet survey data in Sweden and Britain from five 'waves', 2005, 2007, 2009, 2011 and 2013, in order to examine whether the population of non-users had decreased in size but had become more concentrated in vulnerable groups, such as people with disabilities. Analysis of data from Britain revealed that those who reported a disability were more likely to be offline than those who did not report disability-related problems in 2007, 2011 and 2013, and that in 2013, those who reported a disability were twice as likely to be ex-users. Data from Sweden revealed that disability (measured in 2007, 2011 and 2013) was not significantly related to non-use in 2007, but in 2011 those who reported a disability were more than three times more likely to be non-users and 2.5 times more likely to be offline in 2013; disabilities were strongly related to ex-use only in 2011 but not in 2013.

Differences among different disability groups

Although the majority of research in the field tends to focus on the differences between people with and without disabilities, some research has revealed differences among different disability groups. It is essential that these differences are understood further since disability is not a singular construct. In the data analysed by Dobransky and Hargittai (2016) disability status was ascertained by asking participants about both their conditions and their difficulties.

Analysis revealed that once socioeconomic background is controlled for, people with hearing disabilities and those who have limited walking ability are not less likely to be Internet users than people without disabilities, indicating differences between these two disability groups and other disability groups. In a Swedish study, Johansson et al. (2021) surveyed 771 people with disabilities about their use of the Internet and perceived difficulties in using the Internet in order to explore digital divides in-between disability groups, and in comparison, with the general population. Overall, the results of the survey revealed that most people with disabilities are lagging behind the general population, in that they have less access to devices; they use the Internet to pay bills less; they use the Internet for online shopping less; they use mobile banking less; and they feel less included in the digital society. Furthermore, when compared to other respondents with disabilities, people with intellectual disabilities reported lower levels of access to smartphones, computers and tablets; more difficulty in using the Internet; lower levels of using online banking and online shopping; lower levels of using a blog or Facebook; and feeling least included in the digital society.

Barriers to digital inclusion

In addition to understanding that inequalities exist, we need to understand the factors that contribute to these inequalities and therefore what can be done to overcome the barriers to digital inclusion. A commonly cited indicator of digital exclusion used to be lack of access to technologies (typically the Internet). This was labelled as a key indicator of the digital divide. However, as theoretical frameworks and research methodologies have evolved, researchers have distinguished between first-, second- and third-level divides (see for example, Helsper & Reisdorf, 2017; Scheerder et al., 2017). The first-level divide relates to gaps in access to technology among groups. The second-level divide focuses on differences in skills and uses of technologies, and the third-level addresses differences in the outcomes of accessing and using technologies. I have argued that there are four major indicators of digital inclusion (Seale, 2022; Seale, 2009):

1. **Access**
   a.   To technology
   b.   To technology-related services
   c.   To technology-literate professionals/support workers
2. **Use**
   a.   Knowing how to use technologies (e.g. digital literacies)
   b.   Gradations of technology use (e.g. infrequent to frequent use, lapsed user)

   c.   Quality of use e.g. best use or meaningful use
3. **Empowerment**
   a.   Being able to exert control and choice over technology use
4. **Participation**
   a.   Being able to participate in society through the use of technologies
   b.   From civic participation (e.g., voting) through to participation in leisure, education and employment

The importance of considering all four indicators of digital inclusion is acknowledged by numerous studies that have identified barriers to digital inclusion for other people with disabilities. In terms of access, the literature has identified three main barriers: availability, affordability and accessibility. Writing in the context of older adults and teleconferencing, Hawley-Hague et al. (2021) identify poor Internet connectivity and the cost of connecting to the Internet as availability and affordability issues, while Bell et al. (2021) write about the lack of available AT in state-funded sectors for deaf/blind children in South Africa. Writing in the context of Sierra Leone, Austin et al. (2021) reported the results of a study which revealed that the poorest people with disabilities, slum dwellers, consistently experienced a lack of access to AT which hindered their ability to participate in formal (e.g. voting) and informal (e.g. collective campaigning) citizenship activities.

In a similar vein, Tofani et al. (2023) highlight the difficulties in gaining access to AT experienced by refugees and asylum seekers with disabilities entering Italy. With regards to affordability, Locke et al. (2022) highlight the difficulties that visually impaired people experience gaining funding from the Australian government to support the purchase of technologies such as smartphones. Lukava et al. (2022) discuss the prohibitive cost of high-tech solutions such as extended reality. Liaaen et al. (2021) identify the technical complexity of websites and apps as an accessibility issue for people with chronic disease.

The cost and poor affordability of some AT is a particularly important barrier to try to address because people with disabilities are more likely to be unemployed and therefore more likely to struggle financially to acquire AT (Baumgartner et al., 2021). Sometimes the cost of AT is policy-related and is in the power of governments to change, for example by changing import barriers and taxes (Bell et al., 2021). The more expensive technologies tend to be specialist or high-tech. In a position paper resulting from the first global summit on research, innovation and education on assistive technology, MacLachlan et al. (2018, p. 456) argued:

> We are living in a rapidly changing world due to the digital revolution that is not only changing the way people live, learn, produce and even think; but also changing decision-making processes, the way information is delivered, problems are solved and policies are developed. This also makes the distinction between high- and low-tech assistive products increasingly blurred and has the potential to reduce price barriers to high tech solutions.

The main barrier to using technology is a lack of digital skills. For example, in the UK, people with disabilities and those with long-term conditions are 23 per cent less likely to have the essential digital skills for life. Furthermore older people with impairments or conditions might be particularly missing out on the benefits of screen readers, dexterity tools and other AT (see Stone, 2021). A typical solution that is proposed for lack of digital skills is training and capacity building. For example, Bell et al. (2021) argue that if an AT service provides technology, they should also provide training. However, there has been very little consideration of or research into what makes successful training or capacity-building (support) practices. This is something I have been exploring in relation to the digital inclusion of people with learning disabilities (Seale, 2022). Other barriers to using technology include attitudes to technology, lack of fit with a person's lifestyle and a lack of motivation (Baumgartner et al., 2021).

For me, empowerment (agency) is an important indicator of digital inclusion. In a study conducted by Salehomoum (2020) about why deaf adults abandoned their cochlear impacts, results indicated that even though most of the interviewees had been involved in the decision-making process and consented to having an implant as children, all eventually decided to stop using their device. One reason for this abandonment was that they had felt pressured by their families or peers as children to have an implant, but once they became adolescents they felt able to exercise their freedom to make a decision themselves. People with disabilities such as those with communication difficulties, learning disabilities, or cognitive impairments such as dementia who rely significantly on the support of others are at particular risk of having decisions about technology access and use made for them rather than with them. For example, Cumming et al. (2014) shared two case studies in which two women with learning disabilities had been given iPads so that they could use them in an Australian research project they were participating in as co-researchers. One of the women shared how she was having difficulties with staff in her group 'borrowing' the device without permission. The other shared how her device had been taken away from her because her family thought that some of the photographs stored in the iPad were indecent. These researchers suggest that these are examples of people with learning disabilities having choices forced on them.

Sometimes technologies can facilitate the participation of people with disabilities in society by facilitating participation in a range of opportunities such as education, employment, and social and leisure activities. For example, Halbach et al. (2022) explore the role of ICT in enabling the inclusion of people with visual impairments in the Norwegian workforce. Interviewees expressed how ICT was vital for participation in the workforce, but there were a number of challenges in accessing and using them. Vaz et al. (2022) investigate the use of interactive technologies to enable people with visual impairments to participate in museum experiences, while Louw (2018) describes the development of a mobile app to enable people with intellectual disabilities in Ireland to participate in social activities. Sometimes technologies can present barriers to participation in society; for example, digital or smart cities that have not been built with the needs of people with disabilities in mind (e.g. Kolotouchkina et al., 2022). This has led some observers to argue that people with disabilities are at risk of further exclusion:

> The on-going digital transformation of social life with digital media and the increasing use of digital media and technologies for teaching and learning open up new opportunities to overcome exclusion. At the same time, new barriers to participation in society and in education are emerging. These can exacerbate the existing vulnerability of individuals or groups, but also create new forms of vulnerability to social and educational exclusion. (European Agency for Special Needs and Inclusive Education, 2022, p. 9)

The complexity of digital inequalities means that often, removing one barrier does not solve the issue. For example, results from a survey of 106 UK support workers revealed that even if the person with learning disabilities had access to technology, there were a variety of barriers to them being able to *use* it including not knowing how to use the technology, lacking confidence to use the technology as well as lacking skilled and knowledgeable support workers (Seale, 2020).

Global inequalities in accessing technology

Approximately 15 per cent of the world's population are disabled and 80 per cent of them live in developing countries (WHO & World Bank, 2011). Furthermore, we know that greater digital inequalities exist for people with disabilities in the Global South, compared to the Global North. Satari (2021) used data from the GSMA Consumer Survey 2020 to explore the digital inclusion of persons with disabilities in seven low- and middle-income countries (LMICs): Algeria, Bangladesh, Guatemala, India, Kenya, Nigeria and Pakistan. Key findings were that: (1) People with disabilities have lower levels of mobile ownership than people without disabilities in all countries surveyed. Bangladesh has the widest gap, where people with disabilities are 55 per cent less likely to own a mobile phone than people without disabilities. (2) People with disabilities are significantly less likely to own a smartphone than people without disabilities. (3) There is a significant disability gap in mobile Internet use. In each of the survey countries, people with disabilities are significantly less likely to use mobile Internet than people without disabilities. (4) Across all survey countries, fewer persons with disabilities are aware of the mobile Internet than people without disabilities. The World Health Organization conducted a survey in March 2021 to assess access to AT among refugees with disabilities in Bangladesh (WHO and UNICEF 2022). Of the 666 survey respondents, about half reported unmet needs for AT. The reported unmet needs increased with age, which was 31 per cent among young and teenage children aged between 2 and 17 years, 51 per cent among people between 18 and 59 years, and 85 per cent among those aged 60 years and older, respectively.

People with disabilities in LMICs face significant challenges in acquiring AT (Raja, 2016). Three particular barriers to digital inclusion for people with disabilities in LMICs are the cost of assistive technologies, lower state funding to facilitate their acquisition and poorly developed AT service delivery processes. For example, the WHO survey of refugees with disabilities in Bangladesh revealed that the public sector and the government were reported as playing a small role in providing (2 per cent) or paying (2 per cent) for assistive products. The main barriers for accessing assistive products were a lack of support (77 per cent of those reporting barriers), product unavailability (44 per cent) and being unable to afford products (31 per cent). Karki et al. (2023) studied AT service delivery in Nepal, India and Bangladesh. Their analysis of series of interviews with policy makers, AT Service Providers and AT Service Users indicated major weaknesses in AT service provision. AT users have very limited awareness about their rights to these services and the availability of AT services, the range of services available is very limited, and eligibility is dependent on medical criteria related to visible and severe disabilities. Karki et al. (2023, p. 8) argue that increased government funding is needed along with a "medically informed flexible social model of AT services" in order to ensure access to AT services for PWD in these countries.

Global policy responses to digital inequalities

It is widely agreed that addressing the digital marginalisation of people with disabilities requires policy interventions in order to drive broader structural changes in society that are maintaining inequalities in access, use and participation. National and international policy instruments have the potential to place technologies for people with disabilities high on health, social welfare, education and employment agendas. In this section I will provide an overview of three global policy instruments: (1) The United Nation's Convention on the Rights of Persons with Disabilities; (2) The United Nations 2030 Agenda for Sustainable Development in relation to eliminating inequalities and (3) World Health Assembly Resolution 71.8: improving access to assistive technology.

Many commentators position digital exclusion and inequalities as a human rights issue and as a consequence turn to the Convention on the Rights of Persons with Disabilities (United Nations, 2006) for indicators that taking appropriate action to reduce digital exclusion is expected of those governments who sign up to the convention (Ågren et al., 2020; Seale & Chadwick, 2017; Borg et al., 2011). Analysis of the content of the Convention on the Rights of Persons with Disabilities (CPRD) indicates that technology is explicitly referred to in seven of its fifty articles (Borg et al., 2011). Seven articles relate to access to and use of technology. For example, Article 4 refers to promoting the availability and use of AT, and to providing accessible information about AT. Article 21 obliges governments to ensure the right to all forms of communication by accepting and facilitating the use of Braille, augmentative and alternative communication, and other preferred means of communication. Just one article relates explicitly to participation. In Article 29, governments are required to facilitate the use of AT for voting, standing for elections, holding office and performing public functions. None of the articles explicitly refer to empowerment. As of May 2022, the treaty had been ratified by 185 countries and signed by 164 countries. However, there is considerable debate regarding its effectiveness in preventing discrimination and increasing accessibility around the world (Koontz et al., 2022). For example, Borg et al. (2011) criticised the narrowness of scope of the CPRD, highlighting that all the articles fail to cover all the key areas of AT, such as production, availability, affordability, information, training and use. In addition, they argue that the CRPD does not appear to give people with disabilities the right to demand necessary assistive technologies at affordable cost from their governments. Smith et al. (2022, p. 4) acknowledge that not all the articles of the CRPD currently refer to AT; however, drawing on a review of literature, they argue that that there is considerable evidence to indicate that assistive technologies could be used to realise each of the fundamental rights that are affirmed in the CPRD.

They conclude: "The findings of this indicative review suggest the centrality of AT to both achieving the CRPD, and to each of the rights outlined within the convention, ultimately calling for further research and dialogue on the topic to inform equitable policy and programming."

MacLachlan et al. (2018) acknowledge that while the general ethos of the Convention is supportive of AT, it is nonetheless rather vague. They noted that many states that have reported to the Committee of the Convention have not made reference to AT within their reports. In response to this they suggest that states should be required to submit an additional statement which comments specifically on AT and that such a statement would help in the development of national AT policies. Goggin et al. (2019) add further criticism by arguing that the CPRD fails to acknowledge diversity and in doing so ignores inequalities experienced by particular groups of people with disabilities, for example people with cognitive impairments such as those with intellectual and developmental disabilities. Weaknesses such as this lead Goggin et al. (2019, p. 291) to conclude that the implementation of the CRPD is a "work in progress". This may explain why the Coleman Institute for Cognitive Disabilities, based in the US, has created their own declaration of the rights of people with intellectual impairment to access technology.[1]

The 2030 Agenda for Sustainable Development (adopted by all United Nations Member States in 2015) and its 17 Sustainable Development Goals (SDGs) pledges to 'leave no one behind' including people with disabilities.[2] The agenda is, however, vaguer than the CPRD, in relation to the specific role that assistive technologies can play. There is just a brief, very general reference to how information and communication technologies can reduce the digital divide. Perhaps in recognition of this relative silence, Tebbutt et al. (2016, p. 4) drew on research literature to illustrate how the achievement of each of the 17 SDGs could be facilitated by the use of assistive products. They argued that:

> Attempting to achieve the SDGs without appropriate population-level access to assistive products would not only be inherently discriminatory but would also negate the fundamental principle of equity underscored in each goal. In particular people with functional difficulties who need access to assistive technology to be able to equally contribute to reaching the goals in an equitable manner.

However, the 2018 UN Flagship Report on Disability and Development, *Realization of the Sustainable Development Goals by, for and with persons with disabilities*, reported that the status of people with disabilities lagged behind in relation to most SDGs and that lack of access to AT was one of the significant barriers.[3]

In 2018, The World Health Assembly, the decision-making body of the World Health Organization, published the Seventy-first World Health Assembly Resolution 71.8 entitled *Improving access to assistive technology*. It urged Member States to develop, implement and strengthen policies and pro-grammes to improve access to AT, and the WHO secretariat to produce a global report on effective access to AT (WHO, 2018). In 2022, the WHO and UNICEF published a Global Report on Assistive Technology. The report is underpinned by a conviction that: "Access to assistive technology empowers and enables individuals and communities and is a key pre-condition for realization of the Convention on the Rights of Persons with Disabilities and achievement of the Sustainable Development Goals. Put simply, assistive technology is a life changer" (WHO & UNICEF, 2022, p. vii).

The Global Report on Assistive Technology also calls for concrete actions to improve access to AT globally, and recognises AT as both a means to, and an end itself, in the achievement of rights of persons with disabilities (Smith et al., 2022). The report also highlights initiatives that the WHO have undertaken to support Member States including helping Member States develop frameworks that guide planning and implementation of priority interventions and pro-viding resources, such as the WHO Rapid Assistive Technology Assessment tool, which supports the collection of data regarding AT and AT demand/supply situations. The report also anticipates that there will be considerable variations in how countries design and realise AT policies and programmes to address the needs of their populations and that existing national disability or AT-related legislation could be leveraged and integrated into these policies.

While turning to national legislation may seem logical there is much evidence to indicate that relevant legislation, such as that focused on digital accessibility, is currently problematic. The legislation tends to adopt an administrative model of disability, requiring people with disabilities to be formally assessed, using criteria and processes that have been accused of de-humanising people with disabilities. There are not always agreements as to what standards leg-islation should point to in order to set a benchmark for what is considered acceptable and legal and what is considered unacceptable and legal. In addi-tion, such legislation frequently relies on people with disabilities to identify and communicate breaches in law, but even when breaches are reported, governments do not always punish the breaches or enforce the law (see for example, Seale, 2013). There may be a role for researchers in national and international law to examine the extent to which integrating AT policies with related legislation drives the implementation of legislation as much as it drives the implementation of policy.

In order to fill policy gaps, MacLachlan et al. (2018, p. 463) argue that there is a need for evidence-based policy making, where policy is informed by short-term and long-term evidence that is provided by a variety of stakeholders and sources and not restricted to what might be considered strictly scientific standards. One of the challenges for researchers therefore is to provide the kind of evidence that policy makers need:

> Research funding may prioritize "magic bullet" interventions, that would reduce or remove the need for political choice; the scientific method may narrow focus on simplified and controllable variables, while policy makers seek solution to complex problems; "the evidence" may be interpreted selectively, or differently by policy makers; who may need to make decisions quickly amidst uncertainty; need to make decisions, the consequences of which may take years to unfold and which are influenced by other factors.

Capturing and Understanding the Outcomes of Technology Use

The measurement of the outcomes of technology use is argued to be a global challenge. For example, Layton et al. (2022a) argue that if the impact of AT is not captured, then service providers and AT professionals will not know what or how to improve. They describe how the Global Alliance of AT Organisations, GAATO, brought global stakeholders together to articulate the challenges related to outcome and impact measurement as a first step to finding solutions. This resulted in the identification of a longlist of 39 grand challenges, which were condensed into a shortlist of six: (1) measuring need, (2) documenting inputs, (3) measuring outcomes, (4) impacts, (5) sharing data and (6) informing policy. The authors conclude that outcome measurement is the responsibility of each and every AT stakeholder, including users, practitioners, funders, suppliers, educators and researchers. In this section I will consider five particular challenges for researchers in relation to capturing and understanding the outcomes of technology use:

1. Capturing outcomes at all relevant levels;
2. Using both quantitative and qualitative data to capture a range of functional and non-functional outcomes;
3. Capturing the impact of AT over time;
4. Understanding why impact may or may not have occurred;
5. Capturing outcomes that are important to the AT user.

Capturing outcomes at all relevant levels

My analysis of the GAATO (2022) longlist of 39 grand challenges suggests that we are not currently capturing outcomes at all relevant levels: the AT user level, the AT service level and the AT funder or commissioner level (see Table 2.1). We need to adequately capture outcomes at the AT user level in order to identify their strengths; understand the difficulties and barriers they are experiencing; inform service intervention; and understand the impact of the AT, particularly the impact over time.

We need to get better at capturing AT service level outcomes in order to monitor and benchmark service delivery and understand the strengths and weaknesses of AT services. Currently there are just a handful of service-focused outcome measures. For example, The Quebec User Evaluation of Satisfaction with Assistive Technology instrument includes four items that measure user satisfaction with service delivery, repairs and service of the device, professionalism of service and follow-up service (Demers et al., 1996). Another instrument called KWAZO also assesses the quality of AT service delivery from the user's perspective. It consists of seven questions related to accessibility, knowledge, coordination, efficiency, flexibility and influence of the user (Dijcks et al., 2006).

Funders and commissioners of AT services need adequate outcome data in order to establish the benefit of their investments, compare service providers and undertake national comparisons. Policy makers need good outcome data in order to monitor the impact of AT-related policies and make informed policy decisions.

Using both quantitative and qualitative data to capture a range of functional and non-functional outcomes

In AT research the impact of a newly developed AT is typically demonstrated through the use of controlled research trials. In such trials, the effects of a new intervention, in this case an AT, are compared to those of a standard intervention or a control group (no intervention). Sometimes it is possible to randomly assign people to the different intervention groups (a randomised control trial); sometimes it is not (quasi-experimental or non-randomised). Measurements are typically taken before the intervention (baseline) and at various intervals during and after the intervention. Currently, controlled trials tend to prioritise capturing quantitative data about the impact of technologies on disabled users (Roentgen et al., 2021; Saunders et al., 2021; Wijnen et al., 2020; Eichler et al., 2019). They often distinguish between functional and non-functional outcomes where non-functional outcomes capture additional benefits or impacts and are sometimes positioned as subjective. Examples of secondary outcomes include user satisfaction, quality of life and self-efficacy. These functional and non-functional outcomes are captured through a range of standardised

Table 2.1   Mapping the GAATO longlist of AT outcomes grand challenges to different levels

Outcomes	GAATO longlist of AT outcomes grand challenges
User level outcomes	GC9. We do not have outcome measures which address user needs across settings (i.e. home and work)
	GC11. Existing outcome measures do not adequately address all assistive products
	GC21. Existing outcome measures are not inclusive of a range of client populations
	GC22. It is more difficult to evaluate AT outcomes for a person with more complex needs
	GC25. Existing outcome measures do not adequately capture all stakeholder perspectives on the impact of AT on the life of an AT user in a holistic way, including quality of life, wellbeing and health
	GC26. It is difficult to measure the impact of assistive technology across the lifespan
	GC27. It is difficult to capture outcomes for people living in rural and remote areas, often due to difficulty completing follow-up
	GC39. We do not adequately collect and use feedback on products from AT users
AT service level outcomes	GC5. AT personnel do not have adequate education and/or training in outcomes measurement
	GC6. We do not have measures to evaluate the skills of AT personnel, including competency in outcomes measurement.
	GC7. We do not integrate clinical experience and expertise well into outcomes measurement
	GC15. In high-income countries where AT is considered a right, we often fail to measure outcomes as there is no incentive to do so
	GC33. Existing outcome measures do not differentiate well between outcomes related to AT service provision vs. outcomes related to the products themselves

Outcomes	GAATO longlist of AT outcomes grand challenges
Commissioners or funders of AT services level outcomes	GC3. We do not have adequate methods to measure cost-effectiveness of AT, including cost-effectiveness across the lifespan and the cost of failing to provide AT
	GC8. Existing outcome measures are not adequate for interdisciplinary use, or in non-health sectors (social services, education, etc.)
	GC16. We do not have methods to measure the impact and potential costs and benefits of emerging and disruptive technologies
	GC18. Existing outcome measures are not standardised or inclusive of different regions, languages and cultures
	GC 19. It is difficult to measure outcomes which are relevant to the perspectives of all stakeholders, including industry
AT policy level outcomes	GC 12. We do not have adequate systems for monitoring policy-related outcomes (e.g. policy effectiveness, economic evaluation)
	GC 13. We do not have adequate tools to measure supply chain impacts associated with standards and regulation implementation
	GC17. We do not have ways to collect, aggregate and share data cooperatively on a local, national, regional or global level
	GC28. We often do not have consistent or standardised baseline data to compare with after the implementation of new programmes or policies
	GC29. We do not have adequate systems to measure population unmet needs
	GC30. It is difficult to measure outcomes consistently across countries with differing income levels, resources and socioeconomic status
	GC32. We do not understand which objective indicators are required for decision-making and policy development

outcome measurement tools, which are typically in the form of questionnaires. Examples of measurement tools for functional outcomes include the Western Ontario and McMaster Universities Arthritis Index (Eichler et al.,2019); the Hip Dysfunction and Osteoarthritis Outcome Score (Wijnen et al., 2020); and the Disabilities of the Arm, Shoulder and Hand questionnaire (Roentgen et al., 2021). Examples of measurement tools for non-functional outcomes such as user satisfaction and quality of life include the Psychosocial Impact of Assistive Devices Scale (Day & Jutai, 1996); the Quebec User Evaluation of Satisfaction with Assistive Technology Instrument (Roentgen et al., 2021); the Short Form Health Survey-36 (Wijnen et al., 2020; Eichler et al., 2019); and EuroQol (Saunders et al., 2021). There are challenges with the development and use of standardised outcome measures that future research could usefully address. For example, while a few outcome measures (e.g. Quebec User Evaluation of Satisfaction with Assistive Technology) have been validated for different languages, the majority have not. This limits the extent to which impact data from different countries can be combined and analysed together to provide valuable information that will inform global policy responses. There is also scant detail in the AT research literature that would help AT practitioners choose between different outcome measurements tools.

In its global consultation on AT outcomes GAATO (2022) identified that existing outcome measures do not value both quantitative and qualitative data. Some current research studies are starting to capture both quantitative and qualitative outcome data (Dinesen et al., 2022; Hodges et al., 2020; Allin et al., 2020). For example, in evaluating the feasibility and potential impact of a web-based self-management programme for individuals with spinal cord injury, Allin et al. (2020) used a range of outcome measures: the University of Washington Self-Efficacy Scale, the Personal Health Questionnaire Depression Scale, the Spinal Cord Injury Secondary Conditions Scale and the Spinal Cord Injury Quality of Life Resilience Scale. In addition, they interviewed participants. Although they give no details on what questions were asked, Allin et al. (2020) claim that the results from the interviews confirmed and expanded on the quantitative data. For example, they confirmed that participants had made changes to their diet that could be linked to the information contained within the web-based programme. The interviews also highlighted other key factors that the outcome measures did not necessarily pick up, such as the importance of the coach (who was coaching online as opposed to face to face). There is a need for more mixed-method studies like this in order to provide a more holistic picture that captures more of the complexities of the impact of technologies on people with disabilities.

Capturing the impact of AT over time

When AT providers and professionals provide and prescribe AT, they need to know not just that the AT will have an impact, but also, that this impact will be sustained over a prolonged period of time. However, GAATO (2022) identified that it is currently difficult to measure the impact of AT across the lifespan. Controlled research trials can provide evidence that an impact is likely to occur. We need longitudinal studies to tell us if that impact endures. However, longitudinal and follow-up studies are currently rare because they are expensive, often complex and difficult to get funded. One rare example is that conducted by Bäck et al. (2023) who conducted a five-year follow-up study in Sweden of dyslexic students' experiences in using AT to support written language skills. The original controlled trial investigated the effects of assistive technologies (audio books, text to speech and speech to text) on reading or listening to texts (and producing texts) and the motivation for schoolwork during 2014–2017 for a group of students with reading and writing disabilities or dyslexia compared to an age-matched control group receiving treatment as usual. Five years later, a follow-up study was conducted in which nine of the original participants were interviewed about their long-term experiences of using AT in school. The results revealed that their use of AT in the classroom was influenced by their dyslexia acceptance and AT attitudes. Students' understanding of how and why to use AT appeared to limit the development of meaningful strategies. In a systematic review of the literature relating to the implementation of welfare technology for older people, people with disabilities and informal caregivers, one of the conclusions that Borg et al. (2023) drew was that there was a need for more longitudinal studies that could capture how changes in a personal context, such as changes in needs, activities and health status, as well as social contexts (e.g. support available), affected the use and impact of technologies.

Understanding why impact may or may not have occurred

The disability and technology research community has provided valuable information about the existence of digital inequalities and the factors that contribute to those inequalities. In interpreting these data it is clear that the causes of digital inequalities are complex. We know therefore, that simply providing people with disabilities with AT will not necessarily guarantee a positive impact. We do, however, need to increase our understanding of why AT does or does not have an impact. This will require us to invest in more qualitative studies. In order to demonstrate the value of such studies I will shine a spotlight on qualitative research studies that have illuminated the impact of mobility-related AT on the identity of people with physical disabilities.

In a study that sought to examine whether and how 'assistive activity technologies' such as adjusted bikes or modified wheelchairs were used as symbolic expressions of identity by people with physical disabilities, Pedersen et al. (2019) employed semi-structured, in-depth interviews. The interviews covered a range of topics such as the AT allocation process and user involvement, technology and function, identity and personal preferences, social interaction and physical activity. The results revealed that the assistive activity technology provided people with disabilities the opportunity to show themselves from a positive perspective in recognisable and commonly valued activities in society.

Jang et al. (2020) explored the identity development of motorised mobility scooter users. They conducted semi-structured interviews with 20 motorised mobility scooter users. Some of the scooter users reported how the people they interacted with when using the scooter inaccurately assumed that they were less physically or cognitively able than they actually were, simply because they were using a scooter. They concluded that using a motorised mobility scooter may negatively affect how users are perceived by others and themselves.

In order to examine how the introduction of powered mobility impacted the disability identity of children, Feldner (2019) employed an ethnographic approach involving in-depth interviews and field observations of two children and their families. One child had received a traditional powered wheelchair and the other had received an adapted mobility toy. In comparing and contrasting these two case studies, Feldner concluded that identity development of the two children throughout the provision process was influenced by a range of factors including: caregiver perceptions of disability (positive vs. negative), aesthetics and function (medical vs. adventure) and perceived intent of the devices (an opportunity for freedom vs. prolonging need for undesired mobility equipment). Feldner concluded that these findings highlight the varied dynamics and spheres of influence this transaction may have on the developing identity of children with disabilities, which may ultimately help inform future models of provision and rehabilitation practices.

Capturing outcomes that are important to the AT user

One of the longlisted grand challenges that GAATO (2022) identified was that existing outcome measures do not adequately capture all stakeholder perspectives on the impact of AT on the life of an AT user in a holistic way, including quality of life, wellbeing and health. Writing in the context of children and adolescents with disabilities, Beckett et al. (2023) proposed that AT outcome measures need to be re-evaluated in order to address this challenge. They argued that current AT outcomes are adult-centric and do not capture a child's experience and the outcomes that are important to a child. I would extend this argument to suggest that most AT outcomes are rehabilitation-centric, having been designed mostly by rehabilitation researchers with rehabilitation and AT services in mind. In order to address this bias we need to involve AT users in the design of new user-centric outcome measures. However, before we can do this, we need to get our house in order in relation to user-centric R&D methods. In Chapter 9, I will examine in more detail how the disability and technology community currently understands, implements and evaluates user-centric methods such as participatory design and user-centred design.

What should be researched in the future?

In considering the topics or issues that should be researched in the future, the obvious place to start would be the design, provision and impact of new technologies. However, in this section I will argue that there is also a need to research the history of technology design, provision and use.

The Design, Provision and Impact of New Technologies

It is perhaps not surprising that when most stakeholders in the field make recommendations for the future, they identify the need to develop new technologies. For example, the WHO and UNICEF (2022, p. xiv) *Global Report on AT* talks of the need to "transform the existing product range and develop new products utilizing emerging technologies". However, there is a need for care and caution in how we understand the concepts of new and emerging technologies. For example, in a review of patenting and AT trends from 1998 to 2019, the World Intellectual Property Organisation (2021) observed that all emerging assistive technologies utilised enabling technologies such as AI, the Internet of Things and Brain-Computer Interface. However, their data also showed that these emerging assistive technologies were not replacing old or conventional assistive technologies, they were complementing them.

Sometimes researchers believe that new means state-of-the-art, high-tech technologies (Kim et al., 2022) that have never been seen or used before. It is important to acknowledge, however, that new and emerging can simply mean updated, viable or applied differently. For example, in reviewing design studies published between 2018 and 2023 I identified three kinds of technologies that are currently being developed: Standard Mainstream Technologies (see Table 2.2); Advanced Mainstream Technologies (see Table 2.3) and Specialist Technologies (see Table 2.4). All of them are relatively old technologies in that we will have heard of them before. The novelty is in the fact that some are being applied in different contexts (e.g. AI), some are having their capabilities extended or updated in some way (e.g. video games) and others have taken a long time to develop into viable technologies from initial ideas regarding what could be possible (e.g. Brain-Computer Interface and eye-gaze technology).

Table 2.2   Examples of Standard Mainstream Technologies currently being developed

Standard Mainstream Technologies		
Technology	Example studies	Context
Smartphones and associated mobile apps	Huang et al. (2022) Taiwan Visual impairment	Developing mobile technology to support visually impaired pedestrians to cross the road safely
	Alanazi (2022) Saudi Arabia People with intellectual disabilities	Focus group discussions with people with intellectual disabilities about their benefits and barriers of using mobile apps in overcoming difficulties with travel
Tablets	Gibson et al. (2019) United Kingdom Adults with mild learning disabilities	Assessing the feasibility of using tablet technologies to support communication between General Practitioners and patients with mild learning disabilities
	Butt et al. (2020) Pakistan Children with attention deficit hyperactivity disorder (ADHD)	Evaluating the acceptability of a tablet app designed to support the learning of children with ADHD
Wearable technologies (e.g., smart watches)	Koumpouros (2021) Greece Autism spectrum disorder (ASD)	Designing and assessing a wearable technology that supports location monitoring, communication and scheduling of activities for children with ASD
	Jubril and Segun (2021) Nigeria Visual impairment	Designing and assessing wearable technology that will support visually impaired people to avoid obstacles when walking on pathways
Video or teleconferencing	Ochoa et al. (2021) United States Spinal cord injury (SCI)	Determining the feasibility of videoconferencing in promoting increased physical activity for people with SCI
	Allegue et al. (2022) Canada Stroke survivors	Determining the feasibility of using teleconferencing with stroke patients to support and monitor their use of a virtual rehabilitation exercise programme

Standard Mainstream Technologies

Technology	Example studies	Context
The Internet	Hodges et al. (2020) Australia Low back pain	Design and evaluation of a website that aims to provide educational resources for people with Low Back Pain
	Beentjes et al. (2020) The Netherlands Mild dementia or cognitive impairment	Evaluation of the feasibility and impact of a web-based app that aims to help people with mild dementia/mild cognitive impairment (MCI) and their caregivers to find user-friendly apps
Social media	Williams and Gibson (2020) United Kingdom Learning disabilities	Design of a safe social media platform for people with learning disabilities
	Morrow et al. (2021) United States Traumatic brain injury	Examining how people with traumatic brain injury use social media to decrease their social isolation
Video games	Hernandez et al. (2021) Canada Cerebral palsy	Exploring the effectiveness of interactive video games and haptic feedback in improving the arm function of children with cerebral palsy
	Thirumalai et al. (2018) United States Mobility impairment	Designing and evaluating the usability of adapted version of the Wii Fit Balance Board and associated 'exergames' for people with mobility impairments

I am not arguing that we don't need new technologies, rather I am suggesting that sometimes what may be important is to improve existing technologies that present unnecessary challenges or barriers for people with disabilities. A good example of this is the need to improve the usability and accessibility of cybersecurity methods that authenticate users' identities. Furnell et al. (2021, p. 197) argue that:

> Although technology has evolved immensely over the past few decades, reducing the digital divide, authentication methods have changed very little. Authentication is the forefront of securing users' information, services and technology, yet for many it still poses issues in terms of usability and security, due to specific characteristics of different disabilities.

Table 2.3   Examples of Advanced Mainstream Technologies currently being developed

Advanced Mainstream Technologies		
Technology	Example studies	Context
Smart homes	Salai et al. (2021) United Kingdom Learning disabilities, autism or dementia	Studying user perceptions of the value of a system that enables users who have difficulties using voice-based personal assistants to send smart home control home commands
	Moon et al. (2022) South Korea Physical disabilities	An initial evaluation of the effectiveness of a smart home-based modification programme that can be used wirelessly, using Bluetooth, Wi-fi or Zigbee
Artificial intelligence (AI)	Dinesen et al. (2022) Denmark Dementia	Exploration of a how a social robot that uses artificial intelligence and sensor technology interacts with people with dementia
	Tanabe et al. (2023) Japan Profound and multiple intellectual disabilities	Evaluation of an emotion recognition system based on AI using physiological and motion signals.
Internet of Things (IoT)	Jia et al. (2018) China Deaf people	Exploring the extent to which the Internet of Things can support prototypes and product design of vehicles for deaf drivers
	Koppuravuri et al. (2020) India Hearing or speech impairment	Proposing an IoT project which converts hand gestures into synthesised textual format and has the potential to support communication
Virtual reality (VR)	Griffin et al. (2020) United States Chronic pain	Outlining the initial development and implementation of a virtual reality programme designed to help children manage their chronic pain
	Harris et al. (2022) UK Learning disabilities	Using co-design methods to explore the potential applications of VR for people with learning disabilities

Advanced Mainstream Technologies		
Technology	Example studies	Context
Augmented reality (AR)	Miundy et al. (2019) Malaysia Dyscalculia	Conducting initial analysis for Systems Requirement Specifications that can be used to design and develop a visual-based fusion technology AR application for learners with dyscalculia
	LaPiana et al. (2020) United States Stroke	Assessing the acceptability of a smart phone-based AR game as part of stroke rehabilitation for patients with loss of upper limb function

In outlining a global priority research agenda for improving access to high-quality affordable AT, the World Health Organization (2017) identified the need for evidence of what constitutes effective and efficient approaches to AT provision. In response, much of the current research in the field of AT provision has focused on studying and describing the strengths and weaknesses of national AT systems with a view to identifying successful, replicable models of provision and support. For example, Smith et al. (2020) surveyed representatives of key stakeholder organisations in Malawi to gather information regarding AT product and service provision. Key stakeholders included organisations of persons with disabilities, civil service organisations, academic organisations and government ministries who were collaborating to integrate AT into policy and develop a priority assistive products list for Malawi. Results indicated that not all products on the priority list were being provided by organisations; there was a reliance on donor-driven assistive products and a limited number of services available to those who require assistive products. Smith et al. (2020, p. 4) conclude that coordinated AT delivery and service provision is required at a national level which is "sustainable and inclusive and is based on the identified needs of the Malawian population".

Karki et al. (2022) conducted a qualitative exploratory study in order to describe the processes of AT service delivery in Bangladesh, India and Nepal. They interviewed policy makers, AT service providers and AT service users. Their results indicated that improvements to the service delivery processes were needed, requiring a more holistic approach to looking at the process of AT service delivery, from first contact right through to follow-up and device maintenance, with a single door service delivery system, free of cost at the point of service, recommended in these countries. The need for greater coordination is reinforced by WHO and UNICEF (2022) who provide a case study of AT provision in Norway highlighting two key components that they consider important: firstly, collaboration between government departments,

Table 2.4   Examples of Specialist Technologies currently being developed

Specialist Technologies		
Technology	Example studies	Context
Alternative and Augmentative Communication Aids (AACs)	Calmels et al. (2021) France Multi-disabled users	Describing the processes and tools used to co-design AACs for multi-disabled users living in specialised care homes
	Singh et al. (2023) Malaysia Complex communication needs	Exploring how satisfied children with complex communication needs and their parents were with their AAC
Eye-gaze technology	Jeevithashree et al. (2021) India Severe speech and motor impairment	Designing a virtual English keyboard that can automatically adapt to reduce eye-gaze distance
	Hsieh et al. (2022) Taiwan Severe motor and communication needs	Examining the impact of eye-gaze technology on computer use and participation of children with complex needs
Brain–Computer Interface (BCI)	Branco et al. (2021) The Netherlands Locked-in syndrome	Exploring the opinions of individuals with locked-in syndrome, caregivers and researchers regarding what applications users like to control with BCI
Social and care robotics	Maier et al. (2021) Germany Amyotrophic lateral sclerosis	Examining the acceptability of a using a robot arm
	Mitchell et al. (2021) Australia Autism spectrum disorder	Exploring how interacting with a social humanoid robot can support the learning of adults with ASD

professionals, organisations of people with disabilities, manufacturers and research partners; secondly, how specialists work at the national level with rare or complicated needs while generalists work at municipal level with frequent or simple needs. In considering a research agenda for the next ten years, it is likely that more research will be needed in order to satisfactorily address the call by the World Health Organization for more evidence, particularly in relation to impacts, outcomes and quality standards.

The History of Technology Design, Provision and Use

Envisaging a new disability and technology research agenda requires us to imagine the future. It is my contention that in order to imagine the future, we need to understand the past. In particular we need to: (1) understand why some technologies failed, (2) learn from experience and (3) understand how AT designs, processes and services have evolved over time.

Understanding why some technologies fail

Although she was not writing in the context of disability, Light (2001, p. 726) argued that a historical examination of the different ways in which the problem of access to technology has been constructed is needed in order to understand the failure of technologies to reduce the digital divide. Light stated: "A goal for educators should be to reduce the chance that future scholars will look at current efforts to close the digital divide and ask, with the benefit of their historical distance, how could they possibly have thought that?"

In an examination of the history of technology for people with learning disabilities, I discussed three examples of technologies that had failed to live up to their hype: the Carba Linguaduc system, Teaching Machines and Integrated Learning Systems (Seale, 2022). Reasons for their failure were varied but included: being expensive, not being adopted by government provision schemes, lack of evidence of their effectiveness and a failure to convince teachers of their value. Most, if not all, of these barriers still exist today, which suggests new technologies will also run the risk of failure. Learning from failures such as those I identified in my study will require interdisciplinary research teams. For example, we will need engineers and computer scientists to design the new technologies; economists and business researchers to address cost and marketing issues; AT professions and users to design outcomes that can evidence effectiveness; and psychologists and sociologists who understand the factors that influence AT acceptance. In a review of the history of 'rehabilitation aids for the blind' in Canada between 1947 and 1985, Robertson (2020) presents a case study of the R&D programme of an engineer, James Swail, who worked for the National Research Council. They note that Swail was blind himself and as a consequence underpinned his design work with an 'asset-based' understanding of disability. Although this disrupts the stereotypical portrayal of people with disabilities as passive recipients of the technological innovations of others, Robertson suggests that Swail's prototypes were not developed into commercial technologies because the National Research Council considered them to be unmarketable. They perceived the disability market to be too niche and insignificant to invest in. This history neatly illustrates the complexities of digital inequalities and how fixing one barrier won't necessarily solve all the problems. In this example, the involvement of people with disabilities in the design of AT is not sufficient on its own to ensure that people with disabilities can access useful technologies.

Learning from experience

Reflecting on past experiences can teach us valuable lessons about the value that is placed by a range of stakeholders on technologies and what is needed to overcome barriers to digital inequalities. For example, reflecting on the approaches that economically privileged designers adopt, Gregory (2018) argues that they reinforce inequalities when working with poor communities by failing to take into account the past achievements of the community and the past lessons learnt. A pertinent current example of the need to learn from experience is current work that discusses what the 2020 covid-19 pandemic has taught us about the value and role of technology and the implications this has for research, policy and practice. Evidence suggests that during covid-19, people with disabilities were disproportionately affected by restrictions in movement and lack of access to health and social care services and were not always able to ameliorate this lack of access through the use of technologies. The pandemic has therefore taught us that digital participation is more important than ever before (Sube & Buehler, 2022). Smith et al. (2021, p. 151) argue: "We have an opportunity to learn from the COVID-19 response to develop more inclusive and resilient systems that will serve people with disabilities more effectively in the future." One particular area that researchers have identified as a focus for more attention is the need for service professionals to enhance their awareness of the range of different technologies available and increase their ability to use them, and to support people with disabilities to use them. Deverell et al. (2022, p. 260) argue: "COVID-19 has created an imperative for technology laggards to upskill." Current research is still seeking to learn from our pandemic experiences, and it is likely that future research will need to continue this. However, there are other global phenomena such as natural disasters (e.g. tsunamis), wars and economic crises that we also need to learn from because of the impact they are likely to have on people with disabilities' access to and use of AT.

A key factor that limits our ability to learn from the past is that a lot of research outcomes, such as project websites and online conference papers that were produced more than ten years ago, can no longer be accessed. For example, the European TELEMATE project (1998–2001) was set up to develop a framework for the knowledge required by professionals working within the field of AT (see Whitney et al., 2011). As part of this work, they produced two example blended learning courses. Initially the digital resources produced for these two courses were made openly available as part of the funding requirements. However, 20 years later, these resources and the underpinning curriculum framework have become lost to the community. The webpages on which they were hosted no longer exist. Given that there is still a need to build capacity and skills across the community, there may be huge benefits to be gained from re-using and adapting older material and resources. Perhaps we have to re-think what being innovative means in our community and whether it always has to mean 'starting from scratch'. Perhaps we need to lobby those organisations that fund research and development projects to embed 'sustainability' into the judging criteria so that there is an expectation that project teams commit to preserving and sustaining the outputs of their research beyond the lifetime of the project (see for example Khan et al., 2009).

Understanding how AT designs, processes and services evolve over time

Two examples illustrate the value of researching the history of AT designs. Kübler (2020) charts the history of brain-computer interfaces (BCIs) and shows how it has taken over 50 years for BCIs to develop from a mere idea to something viable that can support people with locked-in syndrome to live independently. This is important because it helps us to remember that technology development is not always fast and that in the early days, we have to be careful of overpromising what untested prototypes can offer people with disabilities. Stewart and Watson (2020, p. 1196) draw on oral histories and documentary sources to construct a sociocultural history of the ultralightweight wheelchair. In doing so they highlight how it was designed and built largely by wheelchair users and how the emergence of the ultralightweight wheelchair helped to reconfigure ideas about technology and people with disabilities. Stewart and Watson claim this is a "success story for a group who have historically been excluded from design processes".

With regards to mapping the history of design processes, Begnum (2020) tells the story of how computer science has moved away from specialised adaptations and add-on assistive technologies towards designing universal solutions that attempt to cater for diverse user needs. They argue that this move reflected paradigmatic shifts away from a medical model of disability and from reactive accessibility efforts. There are many debates and disagreements about the value and feasibility of Universal Design, but Begnum (2020, p. 3) suggests that these debates are not necessarily problematic, rather they can be seen as "evolvements over time to complement the different societal systems in which we are designing". The suggestion that Universal Design itself will evolve further is an interesting one for future research to consider, given that some stakeholders are not as convinced of its value as Begnum appears to be (see for example Boysen, 2021; Seale, 2017). In another example of researching design processes, O'Sullivan and Nickpour (2020) map out the 50-year history of 'inclusive paediatric mobility' (IPM) design. They conclude that the field lacks a holistic and rigorous reference point to define, measure, assess and improve the impact of the IPM design process. One driver for change that they identify is the need for improved recording and documentation of IPM design efforts.

Suyama et al. (2023) conducted a narrative review of 92 papers in order to chart the history of assistive devices and home modification services in Japan in the last 20 years. They used this review to highlight implications for the practice of health professionals and of the health care insurance system. Their analysis suggested that sufficient co-operation between professionals was important, and that the insurance system was inflexible. Similar studies in other countries might produce equally useful insights which can inform AT practice.

How do we need to research in the future?

In the previous sections I identified some implications for the way we conduct research in the future; for example, the need for more longitudinal and follow-up studies in order to enhance our measurement of the outcomes of technology use or the need to embrace historical methods such as oral histories or documentary analysis in order to learn from the history of technology design, provision and use. In this section I will discuss the call for more involvement of people with disabilities in AT research and development and the implications this has for a future research agenda.

More Involvement of People with Disabilities in AT Research and Development

The need for increased involvement of people with disabilities in AT research and development has been identified by a range of stakeholders. For example, the WHO and UNICEF (2022, p. 17) argued that the assistive technology system needed to be "people-centred":

> People-centred systems also reflect the importance of user engagement and choice, rather than people being regarded as passive recipients of assistive technology. Active engagement in each step along the assistive technology access pathway – and in strengthening the broader assistive technology system – is critical to an individual realizing their rights and goals, and to the progressive realization of assistive technology access.

One example of the active engagement of users and potential users across the components of the assistive technology system that the WHO and UNICEF (2022) offer is the participation of users in the design and testing of products and services. The research and development community has come to a similar conclusion. For example, in a review of patenting and AT trends from 1998 to 2019, the World Intellectual Property Organisation (2021) concluded that increased co-design of assistive products by end users is needed. Frennert (2021) argues that responsible welfare technology research will involve users in the development of new technologies as part of an attempt to democratise the process of research and innovation. Curtis et al. (2022) and Draffan and Banes (2022) argue that technology design projects that involve AAC users in the design of new products will result in innovative designs that have the potential to produce lifelong changes for AAC users. In discussing the results of their study on the use of cochlear implants by deaf people, Chang and Tucker (2022, p. 11) argue:

> our study suggests there is a need to consider the sociotechnical aspects of AT during the development of these devices, rather than post-hoc. Ultimately, this calls for participatory approaches to AT design that emphasize designing with, rather than for users. Tailoring to the needs of the user of AT through user centric techniques, AT designers may be able to better understand and thus, account for the sociocultural and psychological practices and expectations associated with people who have disabilities, and ultimately, co-construct and develop AT that better serves their needs and improves their quality of life.

Drawing on the motto of the disability rights movement: "Nothing About Us Without Us", Koontz et al. (2022, p. 499) acknowledge that there is a lack of representation of people with disabilities in AT research and development roles:

> We can start by encouraging engagement of AT users at every possible stage of AT research and development. We can strive to make AT research processes more inclusive and to make AT user engagement more authentic. Instead of perpetuating the idea of people with disabilities as the 'researched' and scientists or practitioners as the sole 'researchers' we can share ownership with AT users as 'co-researchers' […] We acknowledge that making significant changes will take time and funding, and we strongly believe the investment is worthwhile.

There are, however, significant differences in how different researchers and developers choose to interpret and implement calls for greater user involve-ment in the design of technologies. These differences are expressed in two major ways. Firstly, there are differences in the extent to which people with disabilities are involved in all stages of research and development, from the initial idea, through to designing the study, bidding for funding and collecting, analysing and disseminating the results. Secondly, there are differences in the extent to which people with disabilities have control or influence over the decisions made during the research (Layton et al., 2021). These differences are not always acknowledged or debated across the AT community which can mean that what one researcher considers to be genuine, inclusive user involvement, another researcher will consider to be partial or tokenistic. Future research therefore could make a useful contribution by fully detailing and evaluating the different approaches to involving users and engaging the community in coming to a shared understanding of what the best approaches to involving users are. A potentially useful place to start is by considering the extent to which the 'ladder of research inclusion' proposed by Layton et al. (2022b) could be applied to AT research and development. In their paper, Layton et al. (2022b) reflect on their experience of practising inclusive research across the areas of assistive technology policy, digital information and health access, as well as the co-design of allied health resources. They position the paper as a description of their journey towards shared power in the mechanisms of research production and how as a team of academics and AT service users they assumed roles beyond the binary of 'researcher' and 'researched'. Drawing on Arnstein's (1969) ladder of citizen participation, they conclude their paper by proposing that there are five roles in research production, and that all research team members, irrespective of whether they are an academic or an AT service user, can hold these roles (see Figure 2.1).[4]

Conclusions and preview

In this chapter I have provided an overarching review of the factors that will influence the development of a future research agenda, the kinds of issues or challenges that need to be addressed by future research and how the questions that arise from these issues may need to be answered. The chapters in this book will expand on these issues through more voices that afford greater detail and perspectives on the foundational topics I have presented.

A research agenda for the future will naturally include the design and evaluation of new technologies. In Chapter 4, Paul Whittington and Huseyin Dogan describe the designs they have produced in response to the challenges that people with disabilities experience authenticating themselves or communicating their accessibility requirements through traditional methods, such as Personal Identification Number (PIN) codes or textual passwords. In Chapter 5, Greg Vanderheiden, Crytsal Marte and J. Bern Jordan outline a proposal for an alternate, supplemental approach to accessibility, where an Info-Bot and an

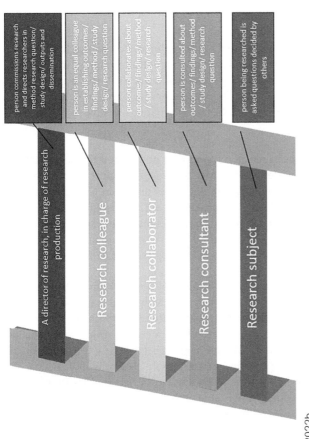

person commissions research and directs researchers in method research question/ study design/ outputs and dissemination

person is an equal colleague in establishing outcomes/ findings/ method / study design/ research question

person collaborates about outcomes/ findings/ method / study design/ research question

person is consulted about outcomes/ findings/ method / study design/ research question

person being researched is asked questions decided by others

A director of research, in charge of research production

Research colleague

Research collaborator

Research consultant

Research subject

Source: Layton et al., 2022b.

Figure 2.1   Ladder of research inclusion

Individual User Interface Generator act as intermediaries between users and interfaces so that the interface adapts to each individual user's needs.

In discussing global policy responses to digital inequalities I identified that a key challenge for researchers is to provide the kind of evidence that policy makers need. In Chapter 6, Robert McLaren, Shamima Akhtar and Clive Gilbert examine in more detail the kind of evidence that policy makers appear to want from researchers by investigating what research the UK government cites in its policy statements on assistive technology.

In discussing the need to measure impact in order to capture the impact of assistive technologies, I identified the need to develop a range of measurement tools that employ both quantitative and qualitative data. In Chapter 7, Dave Edyburn critically analyses the assistive technology service delivery system in order to identify novel approaches to automating assistive technology data collection and analysis.

In this chapter I have argued that we need to understand the past, including learning from our experiences, in order to envisage a future research agenda. In Chapter 8, Rohan Slaughter, Annalu Waller and Tom Griffiths reflect on their experience of building the capacity of AT professionals through the design of a new Masters programme. They draw on this experience to consider what research may be required in the future in order to support the future development of high-quality assistive technology service delivery.

In discussing the call for more involvement of people with disabilities in the design of technologies I argued that future research could make a useful contribution by fully detailing and evaluating the different approaches to involving users. In Chapter 9, I report on the results of a critical review of studies that have involved people with disabilities in the design of new technologies. The review identifies what approaches are commonly used to involve people with disabilities in the design of new technologies; the factors that influence the decisions regarding which design approach to adopt and whether evidence exists to suggest that one particular approach to involving users in design is more effective than another.

Some of the issues and challenges that have been introduced in this chapter will be relatively easy for the community to respond to because of the natural evolution of skills and methods that they already employ. Responding to other issues, however, will push the community outside of its comfort zone, requiring new conceptualisations, new partnerships and new methods. It is this latter challenge that I hope will inspire readers to take action in order to capture the potential of assistive technology for all citizens of the world.

Notes

1. Coleman Institute for Cognitive Disabilities, declaration of the rights of people with intellectual impairment to access technology: https://www.ancor.org/wp -content/uploads/2013/10/technology_and_information_access_declaration.pdf.
2. 2030 Agenda for Sustainable Development. New York: United Nations Department of Economic and Social Affairs: https://sdgs.un.org/2030agenda.
3. Disability and Development Report: Realizing the Sustainable Development Goals by, for and with persons with disabilities. New York: United Nations Department of Economic and Social Affairs; 2018: https://www.un.org/development/desa/ disabilities/publication-disability-sdgs.html.
4. Figure 2.1 is reproduced with kind permission from Natasha Layton.

References

Ågren, K.A., Kjellberg, A., & Hemmingsson, H. (2020). Digital participation? Internet use among adolescents with and without intellectual disabilities: A comparative study. *New Media & Society, 22*(12), 2128–2145. https:// doi .org/ 10 .1177/ 1461444819888398

Alanazi, A. (2022). Smartphone apps for transportation by people with intellectual disabilities: Are they really helpful in improving their mobility? *Disability and Rehabilitation: Assistive Technology, 17*(1), 1–7. DOI:10.1080/17483107.2020.1820 085

Allegue, D.R., Higgins, J., Sweet, S.N., Archambault, P.S., Michaud, F., Miller, W., Tousignant, M., & Kairy, D. (2022). Rehabilitation of upper extremity by telerehabilitation combined with exergames in survivors of chronic stroke: Preliminary findings from a feasibility clinical trial. *JMIR Rehabilitation & Assistive Technology, 9*(2): e33745. DOI:10.2196/33745

Allin S, Shepherd J, Thorson T, Tomasone J, Munce S, Linassi G, McBride CB, Jiancaro T,& Jaglal S. (2020) Web-Based Health Coaching for Spinal Cord Injury: Results From a Mixed Methods Feasibility Evaluation. JMIR Rehabilitation and Assistive Technologies, 7(2):e16351. https://rehab.jmir.org/2020/2/e16351/

Arnstein, S. (1969). A ladder of citizen participation. *Journal of the American Planning Association* 35, 216–224.

Austin, V., Holloway, C., Ossul Vermehren, I., Dumbuya, A., Barbareschi, G., & Walker, J. (2021). 'Give us the chance to be part of you, we want our voices to be heard': Assistive technology as a mediator of participation in (formal and informal) citizenship activities for persons with disabilities who are slum dwellers in Freetown, Sierra Leone. *International Journal of Environmental Research and Public Health, 18*(11), 5547. https://doi.org/10.3390/ijerph18115547

Bäck, G.A., Lindeblad, E., Elmqvist, C., & Svensson, I. (2023). Dyslexic students' experiences in using assistive technology to support written language skills: A five-year follow-up. *Disability and Rehabilitation: Assistive Technology.* DOI:10.1080/174831 07.2022.2161647

Baumgartner, A., Rohrbach, T., & Schönhagen, P. (2021). 'If the phone were broken, I'd be screwed': Media use of people with disabilities in the digital era. *Disability & Society, 38*(1), 73–97. DOI:10.1080/09687599.2021.1916884

Beckett, A.E., Griffiths, M., Khaturiab, M., & Sadaranganib, N. (2023). *Assessing the outcomes of AT for disabled children and adolescents. Is it time for a new approach?* https://aaate2023.eu/wp-content/uploads/sites/26/2023/08/BookOfAbstracts-Prelim .pdf

Beentjes, K.M., Neal, D.P., Kerkhof, Y.J.F., Broeder, C., Moeridjan, Z.D.J., Ettema, T.P., Pelkmans, W., Muller, M.M., Graff, M.J.L., & Dröes, R-M. (2020). Impact of the 'FindMyApps' program on people with mild cognitive impairment or dementia and their caregivers: An exploratory pilot randomised controlled trial. *Disability and Rehabilitation: Assistive Technology, 18*(3), 253–265. DOI:10.1080/17483107.2020.1 842918

Begnum, M.E.N. (2020). Universal Design of ICT: A Historical Journey from Specialized Adaptations Towards Designing for Diversity. In M. Antona & C. Stephanidis (Eds.), *Universal Access in Human-Computer Interaction. Design Approaches and Supporting Technologies. HCII 2020. Lecture Notes in Computer Science, vol 12188* (pp. 3–18). Springer. https://doi.org/10.1007/978-3-030-49282-3_1

Bell, D., Prain, M., & Layton, N. (2021). Assistive technology for people with deaf-blindness in Southern Africa: A Delphi study exploring dimensions of impact. *Disability and Rehabilitation: Assistive Technology, 18*(1), 30–43. DOI:10.1080/1748 3107.2021.1994031

Borg, J., Gustafsson, C., Stridsberg, S.L., & Zander, V. (2023). Implementation of welfare technology: A state-of-the-art review of knowledge gaps and research needs. *Disability and Rehabilitation: Assistive Technology, 18*(2), 227–239. DOI:10.1080/17 483107.2022.2120104

Borg, J., Larsson, S., & Östergren, P-O. (2011). The right to assistive technology: For whom, for what, and by whom? *Disability & Society, 26*(2), 151–167. https://doi.org/ 10.1080/09687599.2011.543862

Boysen, G. (2021). Lessons (not) learned: The troubling similarities between learning styles and universal design for learning. *Scholarship of Teaching and Learning in Psychology.* https://doi.org/10.1037/stl0000280

Branco, M.P., Pels, E.G.M., Nijboer, F., Ramsey, N.F., & Vansteensel, M.J. (2021). Brain-Computer interfaces for communication: preferences of individuals with locked-in syndrome, caregivers and researchers. *Disability and Rehabilitation: Assistive Technology.* DOI:10.1080/17483107.2021.1958932

Butt, S., Hannan, F.E., Rafiq, M., Hussain, I., Faisal, C.M.N., & Younas, W. (2020). Say-It & Learn: Interactive Application for Children with ADHD. In P.L. Rau (Ed.), *Cross-Cultural Design: Applications in Health, Learning, Communication, and Creativity. HCII 2020. Lecture Notes in Computer Science, vol 12193* (pp. 213–223). Springer. https://doi.org/10.1007/978-3-030-49913-6_18

Calmels, C., Mercadier, C., Vella, F., Serpa, A., Truillet, P., & Vigouroux, N. (2021). The Ecosystem's Involvement in the Appropriation Phase of Assistive Technology: Choice and Adjustment of Interaction Techniques. In M. Antona & C. Stephanidis (Eds.), *Universal Access in Human-Computer Interaction. Design Methods and User*

Experience. HCII 2021. Lecture Notes in Computer Science, vol 12768 (pp. 21–38). Springer. https://doi.org/10.1007/978-3-030-78092-0_2

Chang, P.F., & Tucker, R.V. (2022). Assistive communication technologies and stigma: How perceived visibility of cochlear implants affects self-stigma and social interaction anxiety. *Proceedings of the ACM on Human-Computer Interaction, 6,* Article 77, 1–16. https://doi.org/10.1145/3512924

Cumming, T., Strnadová, I., Knox. M., & Parmenter, T. (2014). Mobile technology in inclusive research: Tools of empowerment. *Disability & Society, 29*(7), 999–1012. http://dx.doi.org/10.1080/09687599.2014.886556

Curtis, H., Neate, T., & Vazquez Gonzalez, C. (2022). State of the art in AAC: A systematic review and taxonomy. *Proceedings of the 24th International ACM SIGACCESS Conference on Computers and Accessibility (ASSETS '22).* (pp. 1–22). Association for Computing Machinery. https://doi.org/10.1145/3517428.3544810

Day, H., & Jutai, J. (1996). Measuring the psychosocial impact of assistive devices: The PIADS. *Canadian Journal of Rehabilitation, 9,* 159–168.

Demers, L., Weiss-Lambrou, R., & Ska, B. (1996). Development of the Quebec User Evaluation of Satisfaction with assistive Technology (QUEST). *Assistive Technology, 8*(1), 3–13. DOI:10.1080/10400435.1996.10132268

Deverell, L., Bhowmik, J., Lau, B.T., Al Mahmud, A., Sukunesan, S., Fakir, M., Islam, A., McCarthy, C., & Meyer, D. (2022). Use of technology by orientation and mobility professionals in Australia and Malaysia before COVID-19. *Disability and Rehabilitation: Assistive Technology, 17*(3), 260–267. DOI:10.1080/17483107.2020. 1785565

Dijcks, B.P.J., Wessels, R.D., de Vlieger, S.L.M., & Post, M.W.M. (2006). KWAZO, a new instrument to assess the quality of service delivery in assistive technology provision, *Disability and Rehabilitation, 28*(15), 909–914, DOI:10.1080/096382805 00301527

Dinesen, B., Hansen, H.K., Grønborg, G.B., Dyrvig, A.K., Leisted, S.D., Stenstrup, H., Schacksen, C.S., & Oestergaard, C. (2022). Use of a social robot (LOVOT) for persons with dementia: Exploratory study. *JMIR Rehabilitation & Assistive Technology, 9*(3): e36505. DOI:10.2196/36505

Dobransky, K., & Hargittai, E. (2016) Unrealized potential: Exploring the digital disability divide. Poetics, 58, 18-28. https://doi.org/10.1016/j.poetic.2016.08.003

Dobransky, K., & Hargittai, E. (2021) The closing skills gap: revisiting the digital disability divide. In E. Hargittai (Ed.) Handbook of Digital Inequality. pp. 274-282. Edward Elgar publishing.

Draffan, E.A., & Banes, D. (2022). Augmentative and Alternative Communication Emerging Trends, Opportunities and Innovations: Introduction to the Special Thematic Session. In K. Miesenberger, G. Kouroupetroglou, K. Mavrou, R. Manduchi, R.M. Covarrubias, & P. Penáz (Eds.), *Computers Helping People with Special Needs. ICCHP-AAATE 2022. Lecture Notes in Computer Science, vol 13341* (pp. 477–482). Springer. https://dl.acm.org/doi/abs/10.1007/978-3-031-08648-9_55

Eichler, S., Salzwedel, A., Rabe, S., Mueller, S., Mayer, F., Wochatz, M., Hadzic, M., John, M., Wegscheider, K., & Völler, H. (2019). The effectiveness of telerehabilitation as a supplement to rehabilitation in patients after total knee or hip replacement: Randomized controlled trial. *JMIR Rehabilitation & Assistive Technology, 6*(2): e14236. DOI:10.2196/14236

European Agency for Special Needs and Inclusive Education (2022). *Inclusive Digital Education.* https:// www .european -agency .org/ sites/ default/ files/ Inclusive _Digital _Education.pdf

Feldner, H. (2019). Impacts of early powered mobility provision on disability identity: A case study. *Rehabilitation Psychology, 64*(2), 130–145. https://doi.org/10.1037/rep0000259

Frennert, S. (2021). Hitting a moving target: Digital transformation and welfare technology in Swedish municipal eldercare. *Disability and Rehabilitation: Assistive Technology, 16*(1), 103–111. DOI:10.1080/17483107.2019.1642393

Furnell, S., Helkala, K., & Woods, N. (2021). Disadvantaged by Disability: Examining the Accessibility of Cyber Security. In M. Antona & C. Stephanidis (Eds.), *Universal Access in Human-Computer Interaction. Design Methods and User Experience. HCII 2021. Lecture Notes in Computer Science, vol 12768.* (pp. 197–212). Springer. https://doi.org/10.1007/978-3-030-78092-0_13

Gibson, R.C., Bouamrane, M.M., & Dunlop, M. (2019). Design requirements for a digital aid to support adults with mild learning disabilities during clinical consultations: Qualitative study with experts. *JMIR Rehabilitation & Assistive Technology, 6*(1): e10449. DOI:10.2196/10449

Global Alliance of Assistive Technology Organisations (2022). *GAATO AT outcomes grand challenge consultation.* https://www.gaato.org/grand-challenges

Goggin, G., Ellis, K., & Hawkins, W. (2019). Disability at the centre of digital inclusion: Assessing a new moment in technology and rights. *Communication Research and Practice, 5*(3), 290–303. DOI:10.1080/22041451.2019.1641061

Gregory, S. (2018). Design anthropology as social design process. *Journal of Business Anthropology 7*(2), 210–234. DOI:10.22439/jba.v7i2.5604

Griffin, A., Wilson, L., Feinstein, A.B., Bortz, A., Heirich, M.S., Gilkerson, R., Wagner, J.F.M., Menendez, M., Caruso, T.J., Rodriguez, S., Naidu, S., Golianu, B., & Simons, L.E. (2020). Virtual reality in pain rehabilitation for youth with chronic pain: Pilot feasibility study. *JMIR Rehabilitation & Assistive Technology, 7*(2): e22620. DOI:10.2196/22620

Halbach, T., Fuglerud, K.S., Fyhn, T., Kjæret, K., & Olsen, T.A. (2022). The Role of Technology for the Inclusion of People with Visual Impairments in the Workforce. In M. Antona & C. Stephanidis (Eds.), *Universal Access in Human-Computer Interaction. User and Context Diversity. HCII 2022. Lecture Notes in Computer Science, vol 13309* (pp. 466–478). Springer. https://doi.org/10.1007/978-3-031-05039-8_34

Harris, M.C., Brown, D.J., Vyas, P., & Lewis, J. (2022). A Methodology for the Co-design of Shared VR Environments with People with Intellectual Disabilities: Insights from the Preparation Phase. In M. Antona & C. Stephanidis (Eds.), *Universal Access in Human-Computer Interaction. User and Context Diversity. HCII 2022. Lecture Notes in Computer Science, vol 13309* (pp. 217–230). Springer. https://doi.org/10.1007/978-3-031-05039-8_15

Hawley-Hague, H., Tacconi, C., Mellone, S., Martinez, E., Chiari, L., Helbostad, J., & Todd, C. (2021). One-to-one and group-based teleconferencing for falls rehabilitation: Usability, acceptability, and feasibility study. *JMIR Rehabilitation & Assistive Technology, 8*(1): e19690. DOI:10.2196/19690

Helsper, E.J., & Reisdorf, B.C. (2017). The emergence of a 'digital underclass' in Great Britain and Sweden: Changing reasons for digital exclusion. *New Media & Society, 19*(8), 1253–1270. https://doi.org/10.1177/1461444816634676

Hernandez, H., Poiras, I., Fay, L., Ajmal, K., Jean-Sebastien, R., & Biddiss, E. (2021). A gaming system with haptic feedback to improve upper extremity function: A prospective case series. *Technology & Disability, 33*(3),195–206. DOI:10.3233/TAD-200319

Hodges, P.W., Setchell, J., & Nielsen, M. (2020). An Internet-based consumer resource for people with low back pain (MyBackPain): Development and evaluation. *JMIR Rehabilitation & Assistive Technology, 7*(1):e16101. DOI:10.2196/16101

Hsieh, Y-H., Granlund, M., Odom, S.L., Hwang, A-W., & Hemmingsson, H. (2022). Increasing participation in computer activities using eye-gaze assistive technology for children with complex needs. *Disability and Rehabilitation: Assistive Technology,* DOI:10.1080/17483107.2022.2099988

Huang, C-W., Wu, C-K., & Liu, P-Y. (2022). Assistive technology in smart cities: A case of street crossing for the visually-impaired. *Technology in Society, 68,* 101805. https://doi.org/10.1016/j.techsoc.2021.101805

Jang, S., Mortenson, W.B., Hurd, L., & Kirby, R.L. (2020). Caught in-between: Tensions experienced by community mobility scooter users. *Disability & Society, 35*(10), 1577–1595. DOI:10.1080/09687599.2019.1696749

Jeevithashree, D.V., Puneet, J., Abhishek, M., Singh, S.K.P., & Pradipta, B. (2021). Eye gaze controlled adaptive virtual keyboard for users with SSMI. *Technology & Disability, 33*(4), 319–338. DOI:10.3233/TAD-200292

Jia, J., Dong, X., Lu, Y., Qian, Y., & Tang, D. (2018). Improving Deaf Driver Experience Through Innovative Vehicle Interactive Design. In A. Marcus & W. Wang (Eds.), *Design, User Experience, and Usability: Users, Contexts and Case Studies. DUXU 2018. Lecture Notes in Computer Science, vol 10920* (pp. 257–269). Springer. https://doi.org/10.1007/978-3-319-91806-8_20

Johansson, S., Gulliksen, J., & Gustavsson, C. (2021). Disability digital divide: The use of the Internet, smartphones, computers and tablets among people with disabilities in Sweden. *Universal Access in the Information Society, 20,* 105–120. https://doi.org/10.1007/s10209-020-00714-x

Jubril, A.M., & Segun, S.J. (2021). A multisensor electronic traveling aid for the visually impaired. *Technology & Disability, 33*(2), 99–107. DOI:10.3233/TAD-200280

Karki, J., Rushton, S., Bhattarai, S., & De Witte, L. (2023). Access to assistive technology for persons with disabilities: A critical review from Nepal, India and Bangladesh. *Disability and Rehabilitation: Assistive Technology, 18*(1), 8–16. DOI:10.1080/17483107.2021.1892843

Karki, J., Rushton, S., Bhattarai, S., Norman, G., Rakhshanda, S., & De Witte, L. (2022). Processes of assistive technology service delivery in Bangladesh, India and Nepal: A critical reflection. *Disability and Rehabilitation: Assistive Technology.* DOI:10.1080/17483107.2022.2087769

Kaye, H.S. (2000). *Computer and Internet use among people with disabilities.* National Institute on Disability and Rehabilitation Research. https://files.eric.ed.gov/fulltext/ED439579.pdf

Khan, A.A., Martin, D., & Seale, J. (2009). Sustaining on-line research resources. *Scripted: Journal of Law & Technology, 6*(3), 616–638. https:// script -ed .org/ wp -content/uploads/2016/07/6-3-Khan.pdf

Kim, J.J., Lee, J., Shin, J., & He, M. (2022). How are high-tech assistive devices valued in an aging society? Exploring the use and non-use values of equipment that aid limb disability. *Technology in Society, 70.* https://doi.org/10.1016/j.techsoc.2022.102013

Kolotouchkina, O., Barroso, C.L., & Sanchez, J.L.M. (2022). Smart cities, the digital divide, and people with disabilities. *Cities, 123.* https://doi.org/10.1016/j.cities.2022.103613

Koontz, A., Duvall, J., Johnson, R., Reissman, T., & Smith, E. (2022). 'Nothing about us without us:' Engaging at users in at research. *Assistive Technology, 34*(5), 499–500. DOI:10.1080/10400435.2022.2117524

Koppuravuri, S., Pondari, S.S., & Seth, D. (2020). Sign Language to Speech Converter Using Raspberry-Pi. In V. Duffy (Ed.), *Digital Human Modelling and Applications in Health, Safety, Ergonomics and Risk Management. Human Communication, Organization and Work. HCII 2020. Lecture Notes in Computer Science, vol 12199* (pp. 40–51). Springer. https://doi.org/10.1007/978-3-030-49907-5_3

Koumpouros, Y. (2021). An 'all-in-one' wearable application for assisting children with autism spectrum disorder. *Technology and Disability, 33*(1), 65–75. DOI:10.3233/TAD-200291

Kübler, A. (2020). The history of BCI: From a vision for the future to real support for personhood in people with locked-in syndrome. *Neuroethics 13*, 163–180. https://doi.org/10.1007/s12152-019-09409-4

LaPiana, N., Duong, A., Lee, A., Alschitz, L., Silva, R.M.L., Early, J., Bunnell, A., & Mourad, P. (2020). Acceptability of a mobile phone-based augmented reality game for rehabilitation of patients with upper limb deficits from stroke: Case study. *JMIR Rehabilitation & Assistive Technology, 7*(2): e17822. DOI:10.2196/17822

Layton, N., Smith, R.O., & Smith, E.M (2022a). Global outcomes of assistive technology: What we measure, we can improve. *Assistive Technology, 34*(6), 673–673. DOI:10.1080/10400435.2022.2144690

Layton, N., Bould, E., Buchanan, R., Bredin, J., & Callaway, L. (2022b). Inclusive research in health, rehabilitation and assistive technology: Beyond the binary of the 'researcher' and the 'researched'. *Social Sciences, 11*(6), 233. https://doi.org/10.3390/socsci11060233

Layton, N., Harper, K., Martinez, K., Berrick, N., & Naseri, C. (2021). Co-creating an assistive technology peer-support community: Learnings from AT Chat. *Disability and Rehabilitation: Assistive Technology, 18*(5), 603–609. DOI:10.1080/17483107.2021.1897694

Liaaen, J.M., Ytterhus, B., & Söderström, S. (2021). Inaccessible possibilities: Experiences of using ICT to engage with services among young persons with disabilities. *Disability and Rehabilitation: Assistive Technology.* DOI:10.1080/17483107.2021.2008530

Light, J.S. (2001). Rethinking the digital divide. *Harvard Educational Review, 71*(4), 709–734. https://doi.org/10.17763/haer.71.4.342x36742j2w4q82

Locke, K., McRae, L., Peaty, G., Ellis, K., & Kent, M. (2022). Developing accessible technologies for a changing world: Understanding how people with vision impairment use smartphones. *Disability & Society, 37*(1), 111–128. DOI:10.1080/09687599.2021.1946678

Louw, J.S. (2018). Strengthening Participatory Action Research Approach to Develop a Personalized Mobile Application for Young Adults with Intellectual Disabilities. In K. Miesenberger & G. Kouroupetroglou (Eds.), *Computers Helping People with Special Needs. ICCHP 2018. Lecture Notes in Computer Science, vol 10896* (pp. 454–461). Springer. https://doi.org/10.1007/978-3-319-94277-3_70

Lukava, T., Morgado Ramirez, D.Z., & Barbareschi, G. (2022). Two sides of the same coin: Accessibility practices and neurodivergent users' experience of extended reality. *Journal of Enabling Technologies, 16*(2), 75–90. https://doi.org/10.1108/JET-03-2022-0025

MacLachlan, M., Banes, D., Bell, D., Borg, J., Donnelly, B., Fembek, M., Ghosh, R., Gowran, R.J., Hannay, E., Hiscock D., Hoogerwerf, E.-J., Howe, T., Kohler F., Layton, N., Long, S., Mannan, H., Mji, G., Ongolo, T.O., Perry K., Pettersson, C., Power, J., Ramos, V.D., Slepičková, L., Smith, E.M., Tay-Teo, K., Geiser, P., & Hooks, H. (2018). Assistive technology policy: A position paper from the first global research, innovation, and education on assistive technology (GREAT) summit. *Disability and Rehabilitation: Assistive Technology*, *13*(5), 454–466. DOI:10.1080/1 7483107.2018.1468496

Maier, A., Eicher, C., Kiselev, J., Klebbe, R., Greuèl, M., Kettemann, D., Gaudlitz, M., Walter, B., Oleimeulen, U., Münch, C., Meyer, T., & Spittel, S. (2021). Acceptance of enhanced robotic assistance systems in people with amyotrophic lateral sclerosis-associated motor impairment: Observational online study. *JMIR Rehabilitation & Assistive Technology*, *8*(4):e18972. DOI:10.2196/18972

Mitchell, A., Sitbon, L., Balasuriya, S.S., Koplick, S., & Beaumont, C. (2021). Social Robots in Learning Experiences of Adults with Intellectual Disability: An Exploratory Study. In C. Ardito, R. Lanzilotti, A. Malizia, H. Petrie, A. Piccinno, G. Desolda, & K. Inkpen (Eds.), *Human-Computer Interaction – INTERACT 2021. Lecture Notes in Computer Science, vol 12932* (pp. 266–285). https://doi.org/10.1007/978-3-030 -85623-6_17

Miundy, K., Zaman, H.B., Nordin, A., & Ng, K.H. (2019). Early Intervention Through Identification of Learners with Dyscalculia as Initial Analysis to Design AR Assistive Learning Application. In H.B. Zaman, A.F. Smeaton, T.K. Shih, S. Velastin, T. Terutoshi, N.M. Ali, & M.N. Ahmad (Eds.), *Advances in Visual Informatics. IVIC 2019. Lecture Notes in Computer Science, vol 11870* (pp. 110–112). Springer. https:// doi.org/10.1007/978-3-030-34032-2_11

Moon, K., Lee, Y., Kim, D., & Kim, J. (2022). Smart Home-Based Home Modification Program for Persons with Disabilities: A Pilot Study. In H. Aloulou., B. Abdulrazak, A. de Marassé-Enouf, & M. Mokhtari (Eds.), *Participative Urban Health and Healthy Aging in the Age of AI. ICOST 2022. Lecture Notes in Computer Science, vol 13287* (pp. 267–271). Springer. https://doi.org/10.1007/978-3-031-09593-1_22

Morrow, E.L., Zhao, F., Turkstra, L., Toma, C., Mutlu, B., & Duff, M.C. (2021). Computer-mediated communication in adults with and without moderate-to-severe traumatic brain injury: Survey of social media use. *JMIR Rehabilitation & Assistive Technology*, *8*(3):e26586. DOI:10.2196/26586

National Telecommunications and Information Administration (2002). *A nation online: How Americans are expanding their use of the Internet.* US Department of Commerce, Economics and Statistics Administration. https://www.commerce.gov/ sites/default/files/migrated/reports/anationonline2.pdf

Ochoa, C., Cole, M., & Froehlich-Grobe, K. (2021). Feasibility of an Internet-based inter-vention to promote exercise for people with spinal cord injury: Observational pilot study. *JMIR Rehabilitation & Assistive Technology*, *8*(2):e24276. DOI:10.2196/24276

Office for National Statistics (2019). *Exploring the UK's digital divide.* https://www.ons .gov.uk/peoplepopulationandcommunity/householdcharacteristics/homeinternet andsocialmediausage/articles/exploringtheuksdigitaldivide/2019-03-04

O'Sullivan, C., & Nickpour, F. (2020). Drivers for Change: Initial Insights from Mapping Half a Century of Inclusive Paediatric Mobility Design. In T. Ahram & C. Falcão (Eds.), *Advances in Usability, User Experience, Wearable and Assistive Technology. AHFE 2020. Advances in Intelligent Systems and Computing, vol 1217* (pp. 822–828). Springer. https://doi.org/10.1007/978-3-030-51828-8_109

Pedersen, H., Söderström, S., & Kermit, P.S. (2019). Assistive activity technology as symbolic expressions of self. *Technology & Disability*, *31*(3), 129–140. DOI:10.3233/ TAD-190236

Raja, D.S. (2016). *Bridging the Disability Divide through Digital Technology: Background Paper for the 2016 World Development Report: Digital Dividends.* World Bank.

https://thedocs.worldbank.org/en/doc/123481461249337484-0050022016/original/WDR16BPBridgingtheDisabilityDividethroughDigitalTechnologyRAJA.pdf

Robertson, B.A. (2020). 'Rehabilitation aids for the blind': Disability and technological knowledge in Canada, 1947–1985. *History and Technology*, *36*(1), 30–53. DOI:10.10 80/07341512.2020.1760516

Roentgen, U.R., van der Heide, L.A., Kremer, I.E.H., Creemers, H., Brehm, A.A., Groothuis, J.T., Hagedoren, E.A.V., Daniels, R., & Evers, S.M.A.A. (2021). Effectiveness and cost-effectiveness of an optimized process of providing assistive technology for impaired upper extremity function: Protocol of a prospective, quasi-experimental non-randomized study (OMARM). *Technology and Disability*, *33*(3), 207–220. DOI:10.3233/TAD-210335

Salai, A.M., Cook, G., & Holmquist, L.E. (2021). IntraVox: A Personalized Human Voice to Support Users with Complex Needs in Smart Homes. In C. Ardito, R. Lanzilotti, A. Malizia, H. Petrie, A. Piccinno, G. Desolda, & K. Inkpen (Eds.), *Human-Computer Interaction – INTERACT 2021. Lecture Notes in Computer Science, vol 12932.* (pp.223–244). Springer. https://doi.org/10.1007/978-3-030-85623-6_15

Salehomoum, M. (2020). Cochlear implant nonuse: Insight from deaf adults. *Journal of Deaf Studies and Deaf Education*, *25*(3), 270–282. https://doi.org/10.1093/deafed/enaa002

Satari, A. (2021). *The Mobility Disability Gap Report*. https:// www .gsma .com/ mobilefordevelopment/ wp-content/ uploads/ 2021/ 11/ Mobile-Disability-Gap-Report-2021.pdf

Saunders, R., Seaman, K., Emery, L., Bulsara, M., Ashford, C., McDowall, J., Gullick, K., Ewens, B., Sullivan, T., Foskett, C., & Whitehead, L. (2021). Comparing an ehealth program (My hip journey) with standard care for total hip arthroplasty: Randomized controlled trial. *JMIR Rehabilitation & Assistive Technology*, *8*(1): e22944. DOI:10.2196/22944

Scanlan, M. (2022). Reassessing the disability divide: Unequal access as the world is pushed online. *Universal Access in the Information Society*, *21*(3), 725–735. DOI:10.1007/s10209-021-00803-5

Scheerder, A., van Deursen, A., & van Dijk, J. (2017). Determinants of Internet skills, uses and outcomes. A systematic review of the second- and third-level digital divide. *Telematics and Informatics*, *34*(8), 1607–1624. https://doi.org/10.1016/j.tele.2017.07.007

Seale, J. (2022). *Technology Use by Adults with Learning Disabilities: Past, Present and Future Design and Support Practices*. Routledge.

Seale, J. (2020). Keeping connected and staying well: the role of technology in supporting people with learning disabilities during the coronavirus pandemic. The Open University. http://oro.open.ac.uk/75127/

Seale, J., & Chadwick, D. (2017). How does risk mediate the ability of adolescents and adults with intellectual and developmental disabilities to live a normal life by using the Internet? *Cyberpsychology: Journal of Psychosocial Research on Cyberspace*, *11*, Article 2. https://doi.org/10.5817/CP2017-1-2

Seale, J. (2017). From the voice of a 'socratic gadfly': A call for more academic activism in the researching of disability in postsecondary education. *European Journal of Special Needs Education*, *32*(1), 153–169. https:// doi .org/ 10 .1080/ 08856257 .2016 .1254967

Seale, J. (2013). *E-learning and Disability in Higher Education: Accessibility Theory and Practice*. 2nd edition. Routledge.

Seale, J. (2009). *Digital Inclusion. Research Briefing by the Technology Enhanced Learning Phase of the Teaching and Learning Research Programme.* https://tinyurl.com/4kdjwz6r

Singh, S.J., Ayob, N.M., & Hassan, F.H. (2023). Parents' perception on the use of augmentative and alternative communication by children with complex communication needs in Malaysia. *Disability and Rehabilitation: Assistive Technology, 18*(1), 118–126. DOI:10.1080/17483107.2022.2140850

Smith, E.M., Huff, S., Wescott, H., Daniel, R., Ebuenyi, I.D., O'Donnell, J., Maalim, M., Zhang, W., Khasnabis, C., & MacLachlan, M. (2022). Assistive technologies are central to the realization of the Convention on the Rights of Persons with Disabilities. *Disability and Rehabilitation: Assistive Technology.* DOI:10.1080/1748 3107.2022.2099987

Smith, E.M., MacLachlan, M., Ebuenyi, I.D., Holloway, C., & Austin, V. (2021). Developing inclusive and resilient systems: COVID-19 and assistive technology. *Disability & Society, 36*(1), 151–154. DOI:10.1080/09687599.2020.1829558

Smith, E.M., Ebuenyi, I.D., Kafumba, J., Jamali-Phiri, M., MacLachlan, M., & Munthali, A. (2020). An overview of assistive technology products and services provided in Malawi. *Disability and Rehabilitation: Assistive Technology, 18*(4), 387–391. DOI:10.1080/17483107.2020.1854356

Stewart, H., & Watson, N. (2020). A sociotechnical history of the ultralightweight wheelchair: A vehicle of social change. *Science, Technology, & Human Values, 45*(6), 1195–1219. DOI:10.1177/0162243919892558

Stone, E. (2021). *Digital exclusion and health inequalities: Briefing paper.* Good Things Foundation. https://www.goodthingsfoundation.org/insights/digital-exclusion-and-health-inequalities/

Sube, L., & Bühler, C. (2022). Digital Means for Increased Vocational Participation of People with Intellectual Disabilities. In M. Antona & C. Stephanidis (Eds.), *Universal Access in Human-Computer Interaction. User and Context Diversity. HCII 2022. Lecture Notes in Computer Science, vol 13309* (pp. 400–409). Springer. https://doi.org/10.1007/978-3-031-05039-8_29

Suyama, N., Inoue, K., Kuniya, S., Thawisuk, C., & Kaunnil, A. (2023). History of assistive devices and home modification services under long-term care insurance system in Japan across 20 years: A narrative review. *Assistive Technology.* DOI:10.1080/10400435.2022.2161667

Tanabe, H., Shiraishi, T., Sato, H., Nihei, M., Inoue, T., & Kuwabara, C. (2023). A concept for emotion recognition systems for children with profound intellectual and multiple disabilities based on artificial intelligence using physiological and motion signals. *Disability and Rehabilitation: Assistive Technology.* DOI:10.1080/17 483107.2023.2170478

Tebbutt, E., Brodmann, R., Borg, J., MacLachlan, M., Khasnabis, C., & Horvath, R. (2016). Assistive products and the Sustainable Development Goals (SDGs). *Globalization & Health, 12,* 79. DOI:10.1186/s12992–016–0220–6

Thirumalai, M., Kirkland, W.B., Misko, S.R., Padalabalanarayanan, S., & Malone, L.A. (2018). Adapting the wii fit balance board to enable active video game play by wheelchair users: User-centered design and usability evaluation. *JMIR Rehabilitation & Assistive Technology, 5*(1): e2. DOI:10.2196/rehab.8003

Tofani, M., Iorio, S., Berardi, A., Galeoto, G., Conte, A., Fabbrini, G., Valente, D., & Marceca, M. (2023). Disability, rehabilitation, and assistive technologies for refugees and asylum seekers in Italy: Policies and challenges. *Societies, 13*(63). https://doi.org/10.3390/soc13030063

United Nations (2006). *Convention on the Rights of Persons with Disabilities*. http://www.un.org/disabilities

Vaz, R., Freitas, D., & Coelho, A. (2022). Enhancing the Blind and Partially Sighted Visitors' Experience in Museums Through Integrating Assistive Technologies, Multisensory and Interactive Approaches. In M. Antona & C. Stephanidis (Eds.), *Universal Access in Human-Computer Interaction. User and Context Diversity. HCII 2022. Lecture Notes in Computer Science, vol 13309* (pp. 521–540). Springer. https://doi.org/10.1007/978-3-031-05039-8_38

Whitney, G., Suzette, K., Bühler, C., Hewer, S., Lhotska, L., Miesenberger, K., Sandnes, F.E., Stephanidis, C., & Velasco, C.A. (2011). Twenty five years of training and education in ICT Design for All and Assistive Technology. *Technology and Disability*, *23*(3), pp. 163–170. https://doi.org/10.3233/TAD-2011–0324 https://apps.who.int/gb/ebwha/pdf_files/WHA71/A71_R8-en.pdf?ua=1

Wijnen, A., Hoogland, J., Munsterman, T., Gerritsma, C.L.E., Dijkstra, B., Zijlstra, W.P., Dekker, J.S., Annegarn, J., Ibarra, F., Slager, G.E.C., Zijlstra, W., & Stevens, M. (2020). Effectiveness of a homebased rehabilitation program after total hip arthroplasty driven by a tablet app and remote coaching: Nonrandomized controlled trial combining a single-arm intervention cohort with historical controls. *JMIR Rehabilitation & Assistive Technology*, *7*(1):e14139. DOI:10.2196/14139

Williams, P., & Gibson, P. (2020). CVT connect: Creating safe and accessible social media for people with learning disabilities. *Technology and Disability*, *32*(2), 81–92. DOI:10.3233/TAD-200259

WHO (World Health Organization) & United Nations Children's Fund (UNICEF) (2022). *Global report on assistive technology*. https://apps.who.int/iris/handle/10665/354357

WHO (World Health Organization) (2018). *Seventy-first World Health Assembly Resolution 71.8: Improving access to assistive technology*.

WHO (World Health Organization) (2017). *Global priority research agenda for improving access to high-quality affordable assistive technology*. https://apps.who.int/iris/handle/10665/254660

WHO (World Health Organization) & World Bank (2011). *World report on disability*. https://www.wipo.int/publications/en/details.jsp?id=4541

World Intellectual Property Organisation (2021) *WIPO technology trends 2021: Assistive technology*. https://www.wipo.int/publications/en/details.jsp?id=4541

3. Understanding technology access for people with intellectual disability through Participatory Action Research

Alan Foley

Introduction

The focus of this chapter is the design of technologies with and for people with intellectual disabilities. Person-first language (i.e., 'person with a disability' rather than 'disabled person') is often considered preferable in many professional journals; the idea being that person-first language foregrounds the person, not a 'diagnosis'. Increasingly, disabled activists argue that person-first terminology implies that disability is somehow a diminished aspect of the self, rather than an aspect of identity that is a source of pride. They reject person-first language, and in this chapter, I try to honour this perspective by using disability identity language in general terms. While I use disability identity language in general (i.e., 'disabled person'), I use person-first language when specifically talking about people with intellectual disability and do not use a term like 'intellectually disabled' person. While this usage may seem contradictory, I have several reasons for doing this. While the term 'intellectual disability' describes a condition that some people experience, it is also used as a diagnostic label and as such can connote medicalised, deficit understandings of disability. While some groups have 'reclaimed' a label to identify themselves (e.g., the (D)eaf community, the Blind community, Autistic/neurodiverse folk), many disability groups do not use a specific label to identify themselves because those are often diagnostic labels. In addition, in the United States(US) where I am located, self-advocates with intellectual disability and self-advocacy organisations overwhelmingly use and support person-first language. Finally, I use person-first language when talking about intellectual disability because people with intellectual disability are still often dehumanised and stigmatised. Other terms for intellectual disability (namely the 'r-word') have been and are still sometimes used pejoratively in ways that other disability categories/labels are not.

Intellectual disability is a condition that affects millions of people worldwide and is characterised by significant limitations in cognitive functioning and adaptive behaviour. People with intellectual disability often face significant barriers to full participation in society, including limited access to education, employment, health care and other essential services. Historically, they have been excluded from decision-making processes that affect their lives and have been subject to stigma and discrimination. Despite the ubiquity of many technologies, access to technology for disabled people in general remains a problem; however, there are demonstrated benefits of technology use by people with intellectual disability. For example, adults with intellectual disability often have limited social networks and social capital (Davies et al., 2015), and technology can provide opportunities to connect. A study on the use of Facebook indicates that adults with intellectual disability use Facebook as often as nondisabled users, and social networking sites have the potential to support social relationships and self-determination (Shpigelman & Gill, 2014). Similarly, a study conducted with teenagers who use augmentative and alternative communication (AAC) found a perceived benefit of social media participation and enhanced self-representation and self-determination (Hynan et al., 2015). For many people with intellectual disability, 'technology' and 'assistive technology' are the same. One mobile device, for example, can provide communication support and connect to the Internet; separate devices are not necessary (Foley & Ferri, 2012).

While the research base continues to grow, there still is a gap between the knowledge we currently have regarding technology use in society at large and the use and accessibility of technology for individuals with intellectual disability. This knowledge gap exists in part because there continues to be a divide with regard to the number of disabled people in general who own or have access to technology compared to the general public (Vicente & López, 2010). In addition, mere access to technology does not necessarily correspond to increased use; technology usage among disabled people in general is lower than among groups without disabilities even when both groups own computers (Sachdeva et al., 2015). Finally, in contrast to web accessibility guidelines that comprehensively cover other forms of disability that require the use of certain assistive technologies (e.g., blindness), guidelines for technology that is accessible and useable for people with intellectual disability are incomplete and inconsistent, largely developed through trial and error and not representing evidence-based practice (Friedman & Bryen, 2007).

More specific to higher education and the research context is the scarcity of disabled researchers, especially those with intellectual disability, and the persistence of ableist beliefs of what research is and who researchers are. This can manifest itself in many ways. For example, researchers may use complex language or technical terms that are difficult for people with intellectual disability to understand. They may also assume that individuals with intellectual disability are not able to give informed consent or make decisions about their participation in research.

These attitudes are buttressed by the neoliberalisation of higher education, which intensifies and extensifies what is expected of academics and further limits who is seen as 'able' to generate knowledge. Despite decades of legislation mandating a framework of social justice and human rights for addressing the needs of disabled individuals (Guillaume, 2011) such as the Americans with Disabilities Act (ADA) and Section 504 of the Rehabilitation Act of 1973 in the US, as well as provisions for access to education in the United Nations Convention on the Rights of Persons with Disabilities (CRPD), disabled students remain excluded from and marginalised within higher education (Harbour & Greenberg, 2017). This disconnect between the 'legal' rights of disabled students to access higher education and what they encounter is symptomatic of the ableist and exclusionary history of higher education (Dolmage, 2017). Even as many universities publicly proclaim their commitment to 'inclusivity' they continue to make construction and design decisions that limit access for people with mobility, or select software systems that are not accessible for people who use screen readers. While it is no longer socially acceptable to hold events that are racist or culturally appropriative, overtly ableist service projects in which disability is pitiable and in need of charity (and correction) still appear on campuses in the US. While student athletes are allowed various academic supports and resources, disability accommodations such as extended time on tests are often still viewed as an unfair advantage, or something to be 'gamed' for college admissions by affluent families (Miller, 2019). It is still possible to hear students laughingly calling each other 'retarded' while walking across a college campus.

Similar to how institutions may have policies promoting diversity, equity and inclusion but not be antiracist, policies supporting accessibility are not anti-ableist. Accessibility policies do not disrupt overt and dysconscious ableism. Broderick and Lalvani (2017) describe dysconscious ableism as "an impaired or distorted way of thinking about dis/ability (particularly when compared to critical conceptualizations of dis/ability), one that tacitly accepts dominant ableist norms and privileges" (p. 895).

There is a considerable gap between the knowledge we currently have regarding technology use in society at large and the use and accessibility of technology for individuals with intellectual disability (called learning disability in the United Kingdom). This knowledge gap exists in part because there continues to be a divide in the number of disabled people in general who own or have access to technology compared to the general public and, importantly, because disabled people are not involved in the development process. An approach to address this is inclusive research and design, particularly with regard to engaging people with intellectual disability in Participatory Action Research (PAR). This chapter will describe a participatory approach to technology development with and for people with intellectual disabilities and discuss some of the unique challenges and opportunities a participatory technology development project offers. It will provide examples from a participatory project to develop digital tools to support self-advocacy and community living for people with intellectual disability and investigate use of technology by individuals with intellectual disability (Foley, 2019).

What is Participatory Action Research?

Participatory Action Research (PAR) can be described as a family of research methodologies that pursue action or change and research at the same time, combining action research and participatory praxis. Action research is a way of generating research about a social system while simultaneously attempting to change that system. PAR is participative because change is usually easier to achieve when those affected by the change are involved in the research.

PAR involves academic–community partnerships to identify areas of study, conduct research, interpret results and translate information back to communities for strategic planning and action. PAR is an approach and set of processes that involve a dynamic and sustained collaboration between researchers, constituents with disabilities and community stakeholders, such as policy makers, planners, housing and transportation representatives, and public and private entities interested in expanding opportunities for people with disabilities. PAR can also improve the quality, impact and value of the research, as it is more likely to be used in policy and systems change actions that affect larger groups of disabled people in communities and regions (Conder et al., 2011; Bigby & Frawley, 2010; Oden et al., 2010; Minkler et al., 2008). PAR aims to be emancipatory; increase self-esteem, self-efficacy and empowerment of a community that has historically been exploited and oppressed by research methods; promote social justice; build capacity; disrupt problematic discourses; and be reflective and transform the relationships between the community and professional researchers.

Despite its advantages, it is important to note that PAR also presents challenges, including the need to devote time to building relationships, create and provide accommodations to participate and devise ways to share power over the nature and direction of research. Thus, PAR demands collaboration skills, adequate resources and time to foster and sustain full participation (Hammel et al., 2016; McDonald & Stack, 2016).

PAR is intentionally interventionist by developing interventions (Sitbon, 2018), producing tools (Sitbon & Farhin, 2017), strengthening community resources (Hammel et al., 2016) and decreasing disparities (Beighton et al., 2019; Nicolaidis et al., 2015; Zhang & Dorn, 2013). PAR supports disabled people taking an active role in designing and conducting research (Knox et al., 2000) and can disrupt what has been described as the parasitical nature of a great deal of research activity on disability (Barton, 2005). Centring the lived experiences and privileging the knowledge and expertise of people with intellectual disability, PAR can play an affirmative role in challenging dysconscious ableism. PAR speaks directly to ableist opinions/beliefs about what research is, who can conduct it and who has access to higher education (Dolmage, 2017).

PAR promises to democratise knowledge production and empower marginalised communities by giving them a voice in shaping research questions, methods and outcomes. Additionally, PAR aims to produce research that is directly relevant to the community's needs and can lead to actionable change. In the following sections, I will draw on my recent experience with a PAR project called 'Community for All' to illustrate and discuss the value of employing PAR with people with intellectual disability in order to promote technology access and use.

The Community for All project

Despite decades of advocacy and policy changes, living in the community and having a self-directed life is still not an option for many people with intellectual disability in the US. Thousands of people with intellectual disability continue to live in institutional settings, and many more experience segregation from their communities (Larson et al., 2013). The self-advocacy movement is a broad and diverse collation of people with intellectual disability and their allies. The Community for All project (C4A) was a participatory project funded by a grant from the Administration for Community Living (ACL), in the Department of Health and Human Services, to develop digital tools to support self-advocacy and community living for people with intellectual disability and investigate use of technology by individuals with intellectual disability. By developing digital tools to support self-advocacy and community living with and for people with intellectual disability, the goals of the C4A project were to improve understanding of digital access for individuals with intellectual disability and increase self-advocacy, independent living and community participation for individuals with intellectual disability using web-based and mobile tools.

The self-advocacy movement began in Sweden in the 1960s when a group of people with intellectual disability prepared a list of requests about how they wanted services delivered and what they wanted from their service providers. One of the partners for the C4A project, the Self-Advocacy Association of New York State (SANYS), describes self-advocacy as, "speaking up for yourself. It is making your own choices in life, big and small. It is learning about your rights and responsibilities. It is living the way you want to and respecting the right of others to do the same".[1] It is important to keep in mind that historically, people with intellectual disability have had little or no say in their lives and were often forced to live apart from the community in institutions. People with intellectual disability still encounter discrimination and assumptions that they cannot make decisions about their own lives, and the self-advocacy movement is a response to these attitudes. Self-advocacy includes a wide range of activities that people without intellectual disability often take for granted. For example, self-advocacy might include asking an employer for equal opportunities in the workplace, choosing to have a medical procedure or not to have it, or deciding to paint one's bedroom.

The C4A project team was comprised of self-advocates with intellectual disability, self-advocacy advisors, user experience and graphic designers, university researchers, and graduate and undergraduate students. The overarching design principle for the tools was that people with intellectual disability should immediately and intuitively recognise themselves as the specific audience through carefully researched and designed content, language and graphics.

Phases of the C4A Project

The C4A team used a design and development process drawn from design research for designing the digital tools with specific goals or objectives, testing them, evaluating the results and then refining or adjusting the intervention, in this case refining and improving with members of the target population (people with intellectual and developmental disabilities), as well as other users like family members or support personnel.

At its most fundamental level, design research is about transforming practices in authentic situations (Cobb et al., 2003). Thus, a design study seeks to better understand how an intervention operates in an authentic situation through a process of problem identification, theory development, intervention design, iterative implementation and coordination with participants, feedback, revision, evaluation and reflection.

Design studies narrow the gap between research and practice by conducting research in situ, where hypotheses and interventions are observed, and data are collected in a situated environment rather than a laboratory setting. The benefit of this practice is to advance the external validity and authenticity of 'what works' in an environment where research controls are difficult to transfer to practice (Walker, 2006). The design, development and implementation of the C4A digital tools were conducted using a framework comprised of interrelated and iterative phases (see Figure 3.1).

This process involves several phases in an iterative process: analysis of problems, development of solutions, iterative cycles of testing and refinement, and reflection on design and implementation. This process helped the team integrate the development of the tools rather than focus on discrete 'steps' such as: concept, user interface, user experience prototyping, user-testing and content design. The C4A team was organised into multiple workgroups with each workgroup working on a different tool area and coordinating with the other groups. Each workgroup had designated co-leaders, one being a self-advocate, who shared the responsibility of the co-leader role.

The C4A project developed materials and tools for people with intellectual disabilities and the people who support them. Some of the C4A tools developed included a MemeGenerator, a rider profile (for people using public transportation), and a social media quiz. The MemeGenerator tool was designed to help people engage in social media activism and explore disability identity and pride by creating memes they could share on social media. There were three categories of memes: 1) create your own meme, 2) 'Memes 2 Go' already created and ready to share and 3) a mix-and-match where a user selects an image and then chooses from prewritten text. The Rider Tool was designed to allow users to be proactive in creating a way to share information about themselves with public transportation and ride-share drivers to allow greater understanding of their needs and ways of being. The social media quiz was an interest inventory/quiz

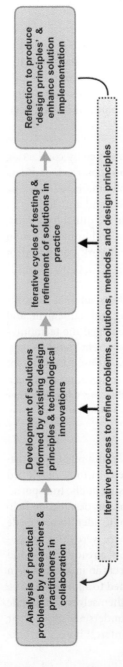

Source: Adapted from Amiel & Reeves, 2008.

Figure 3.1   The design research process

designed to help users find social media platforms that cater to their preferred methods of engagement (text, images, video).

Participatory Perspectives: Logo and Icon Development

An example of the project's participatory and design research approach can be seen in the development of the logo for the project and the icons the team developed to represent the six categories the tools the team was developing fell into. The project team chose to start with these pieces of the project because they were relatively small. The team felt it could get them completed quickly and that developing these representations of the project would help the team develop a shared vision of the project and work together immediately. The project team worked with an undergraduate student designer through several iterations of both the logo and the icons.

While the team was developing the project logo, it also developed icons representing the six topical areas in the C4A project (see Figure 3.2). The team developed these icons with the plan that it would use them on the C4A website and associated apps; however, the icons also give the team a way to differentiate tools and communicate about them internally.

Much of the feedback from the team, especially the self-advocate team, focused on the images associated with the icons. The self-advocates had several conversations about what these images convey and how to convey meaning without words. An early version of the icons featured images (see Figure 3.3) that resonated with the white, female, college-aged designer, but were unclear to some members of our team.

The images chosen by the designer were heavily influenced by mobile and cloud technologies. Community participation was represented by a network node diagram (connections), self-advocacy with a speech bubble (speaking up), families with a heart and digital community with a cloud (cloud-based technologies). The team gave the designer the following written feedback (this was transcribed into an email by a team member while the group was discussing):

1. We like colours and how the icons fit in the middle of the pointer – we think that will definitely work and want to move forward with that element.
2. The one for self-advocacy – we saw that it was a speech bubble, we think that a megaphone would be stronger, or something showing a person's voice.

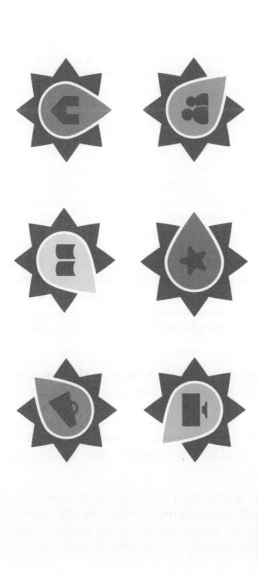

Note: Clockwise from top left: self-advocacy for all; lifelong learning for all; community living for all; digital communities for all; community participation for all; family for all.

Figure 3.2   C4A final icons

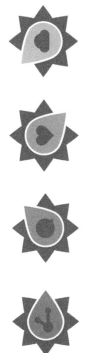

Note: From left to right: community participation for all; self-advocacy for all; family for all; digital communities for all.

Figure 3.3   An early draft of C4A icons

3. Family – the heart alone seems too close to the icons for health apps. Also, many of us do not have 'loving' relationships with family – there might be issues of control, alienation, and so on. One idea is something like those family stickers you see on the back of mini vans and SUVs with the different-sized people and pets. We understand the issues with that representation of 'family' too, but the team feels it is a more recognizable image.
4. Digital – the cloud is too abstract – a smartphone or computer probably is a safer bet.
5. The 'sharing' or 'network node' icon seems too abstract … maybe something with people being connected.

Evaluating the extent to which the Community for All project illuminated the principles and challenges of PAR

The overarching aim of the C4A Project was to involve people with intellectual disabilities as equal partners in the design of digital resources that would be of direct relevance to them. We adopted a PAR approach in order to achieve our aim. In order to convince others that there is value in adopting this approach more widely it is important to reflect on the extent to which we were successful in implementing the principles of PAR and the extent to which we also experienced the challenges of PAR. To underpin these reflections I will use the framework of principles and challenges offered by Balcazar et al. (1998). They articulate the following four principles for conducting PAR in collaboration with disabled people:

1. Disabled people should articulate the problem and participate directly in the process.
2. The direct involvement of disabled people in the research process allows participants to share objective and subjective aspects of their (lived) experience.
3. Participating in PAP can increase awareness among disabled people about their own resources and strengths and help develop leadership skills among the participants.
4. The goal of PAR with disabled people is to improve the quality of life for disabled people.

Conversely, Balcazar et al. (1998) identify some challenges that can arise in PAR projects working with disabled people:

1. Developing participatory relationships can take a long time.
2. Questions about who controls the research endeavour can arise.
3. PAR can be time-consuming and not mesh well with timelines of academe.
4. Participatory research brings unintended consequences.

Reflections on How the Community for All Project Implemented PAR Principles

The four principles of PAR described by Balcazar et al. (1998) were not proposed specifically in relation to the participation of people with intellectual disability in PAR projects. In this section I will draw on comments from team members in order to illustrate the potential applicability of these principles to intellectual disability-focused PAR projects.

Disabled people themselves articulate the problem and participate directly in the process

With regards to their first principle, Balcazar et al. (1998) consider significant participant involvement the most fundamental principle of PAR. There is evidence to indicate that this was achieved in the C4A project. For example, one of the nondisabled members of the C4A project team noted: 'Having self-advocates as part of the teams played an integral role in the development of the tools. Their insight has proven substantial, and their involvement has been nothing short of tremendous.'

The direct involvement of disabled people in the research process allows participants to share objective and subjective aspects of their (lived) experience

One of the C4A team members with intellectual disability observed: 'I feel like I've made some new friends on the way. I've gotten to know people on the third floor [academics and staff at the university] and it feels good to come up to the third floor and know people. The best part of all is that we are trying to make a difference.'

Many of our team members had previously had little or no interaction with people with intellectual disability as reflected by one of the programmers on the project: 'Personally, I have never worked on any kind of project or job with [people with intellectual disability] before ... I have found working with self-advocates as part of the project to be a great opportunity.'

Another member noted: 'Our commitment to being a participatory project is a consistent reminder to me to be sure I am communicating effectively with the ENTIRE team and gives me new perspective on how people use experience and use technology.'

Increasing awareness among disabled people about their own resources and strengths and helping to develop leadership skills

Capacity building is important when conducting PAR with people with intellectual disability and is often more complex than it might seem at first. While there are various different approaches to training and capacity building for research with people with intellectual disability, the approach taken must be reciprocal and must strike a balance between understanding things (the academic agenda) and changing things (the self-advocacy agenda) (Nind et al., 2016). Moreover, Nind et al. (2016, p. 3) observe that "the academic researcher is at an advantage and cannot necessarily expect researchers with intellectual disability to already have research skills".

Our project team included senior and newer self-advocates with intellectual disability, and one of the experienced self-advocates expressed the following in relation to their own personal development: 'It means a lot to be part of the project. My main goal in my career has been to teach others with developmental disabilities how to advocate for themselves ... It is great to mentor young self-advocates and watch them grow because they are the future of the movement.'

A newer self-advocate said about their participation in the project: 'It has helped me learn about other ways of thinking ... It has helped me learn about other people's thoughts and ideas about the disability movement and people that have disabilities.'

Improving the quality of life for disabled people

PAR contributes to an improvement in quality of life by encouraging participants to critically reflect on their living conditions, strengthening grassroots organisations and developing the capacity of the participants to address their own needs. One of the C4A self-advocates addressed this directly:

> Being part of the team for me means working with a diverse group of individuals who have helped me become a stronger advocate for myself and others. In addition, I am truly grateful to have been able to provide my insight so that many others may benefit in the future from my experiences.

What Did We Learn about the Challenges of PAR through the Community for All Project?

Despite its advantages, it is important to note that PAR also presents many challenges, including the need to devote time to building relationships, create and provide accommodations to participate and devise ways to share power over the nature and direction of research. Thus, PAR demands collaboration skills and adequate resources and time to foster and sustain full participation (McDonald & Stack, 2016; Stack & McDonald, 2014; Nicolaidis et al., 2011). Balcazar et al. (1998) highlighted challenges they felt were most relevant to building collaborative relationships between university researchers and disabled people. In this section I will reflect on whether and how the C4A project experienced similar challenges.

The length of time it takes to develop participatory relationships

Gaining entry and developing participatory relationships can take months and may require researchers to establish relationships through volunteer work or other activities with the community. Potential barriers to entry can include identity differences (race, class, disability, age, gender, etc.);perceived and actual power differences, particularly around questions of who controls funding; a previous negative history of the community with university researchers (e.g., misleading researchers); researchers taking an overly directive approach to working with community members; or a lack of pre-existing community ties. A participatory development project by and for people with intellectual disability is very different from a project where 'experts' create specifications, hire developers and build some technology. We were committed to having meaningful participation by people with intellectual disability as well as improving access to and use of technology by people with intellectual disability. When the project began, the team knew it would have depth in content areas (both team members with and without intellectual disability). The campus centre, through which the project ran, had been engaged in supporting community living and participation and self-advocacy for many years and regularly worked with self-advocates in the community. The centre also had long-standing partnerships with self-advocacy organisations. From the start, the team included members with intellectual disabilities who had experience in self-advocacy. It proved more challenging to find people with intellectual disability with experience in any form of technology development. To address that issue, the team decided to recruit several members of the team who were interested in technology and then work with them to build the knowledge and skills the project requires. While the project did have technical staff, their role did not just involve development but also working with other team members in building skills.

Issues relating to who controls the research endeavour

Relinquishing control of the research endeavour can be difficult or raise issues in academic contexts. Because disabled people participate directly in the process, Balcazar et al. (1998) noted that researchers had raised questions about whether PAR can have a role in basic (i.e., lab) research. These researchers considered that PAR can have a role in applied research and that PAR is useful for qualitative studies but less appropriate for quantitative studies where there is the issue of experimental control. Such concerns reflect the beliefs/opinions that relinquishing experimental control is equivalent to relinquishing the research enterprise itself and that some types of research are more valid than others. Moreover, beliefs and opinions that imply some people can or cannot conduct 'rigorous' research suggests that dysconscious or even overt ableism is at play. One approach that our project team took to address this issue was using a co-leader concept to guide sub-groups working on various components of the project. Each sub-group had designated co-leaders, one being a self-advocate, who shared the responsibility of the co-leader role.

The misalignment between PAR and academic timelines

Typically, participatory research takes several years, and this long timeframe can be an issue particularly for those working towards tenure or under other academic pressures. Collaborative projects can typically take three to five years. C4A took five years, considerably longer than other technology development projects the author has conducted. Some of this is due to the nature of a participatory project where we try to have meaningful input from all the team, and some of this is from the complexities of working with people with intellectual disability in a context (higher education for example) that tends to exclude them. Our team spent more time on project management than it might have with a less participatory team. The team's decision-making process was slower than if it were only top-down. It takes time to build consensus, and it was important to document decisions in ways that were relevant and accessible to the entire team (i.e., the group could not solely rely on written documentation and email threads to communicate).

Another factor that added to the length and complexity of the project was that our team had accommodation, travel and facilities logistics to negotiate. Disabled people can have more than one impairment (e.g., being a wheelchair user, having a vision or hearing impairment, having autism, etc.) so as a project team we had to anticipate not just how we could accommodate intellectual disability, but also any other disability the self-advocates might have (and disabilities of other team members as well). The project being based on a university campus meant the team had limited access to parking in general and had to plan well in advance for accessible parking. In addition, finding meeting spaces on a university campus can be challenging, and finding meeting spaces that are accessible that could accommodate our group was an added challenge. At a minimum, our meeting spaces had to be able to accommodate two to three motorised wheelchairs, support staff and other team members.

Technology development teams in general tend to underestimate the amount of time tasks will take and, therefore, encounter moments of 'crunch time', where team members are working late into the night, weekends, or while travelling. All too often projects rely on the capacity and flexibility of team members to absorb such unplanned time. For the academics on our team, this kind of inconsistently flexible time was normal, but other members of our team did not have that kind of 'flexibility' or did not want it. Setting realistic deadlines in this context means considering the life situations and experiences of all team members, not just the members who have a 'traditional professional' background.

The unintended consequences of participatory research

Because PAR projects pursue both change and research at the same time, the effects it can have on its participants and the context can be unanticipated. One of the more positive consequences is that all participants can develop a more critical view of the world and a better understanding of the rights and needs of disabled people. However, it may also lead participants to question/criticise their relationships with researchers and/or sponsoring organisations. Participants typically criticise what is known to them, which may include community organisations or support agencies and possibly what they see as shortcomings of researchers and research process. These types of questions and criticism might be awkward or uncomfortable but are nonetheless important as they are also part of capacity building and self-advocacy. Another unintended consequence is that there may be risk that comes from challenging the status quo. In situations where projects are engaged in advocacy efforts there might be a risk of reprisals from opposing agencies or organisations that might disproportionally affect the disabled participants on the project.

In addition to the challenges that Balcazar et al. (1998) have noted, another significant challenge to conducting PAR in university settings around technology is ableism in higher education and in the technology sector, particularly with respect to intellectual disability. This often manifested as various forms of workplace inaccessibility and institutional lack of response to inaccessibility. Because the project was organised and supported by a university, everyone working for the project was an employee of the university and subject to its employment requirements and expectations. Late in the project, the university made it a requirement that every employee complete a university-provided diversity training. At the beginning of one of our working groups a self-advocate came in very worried about an email they had just received regarding training that was mandatory and due by the beginning of the following week in order to remain employed. As a team we were able to drop everything and, on the spot, offer an accessible version of the training. Another example of institutional inaccessibility during the project was a shift in timesheet format and submission process midway through the project. When the project began, timesheets were paper-based, and the team came up with an accessible support system for self-advocates to complete timesheets. When the university switched from paper timesheets to an online system, many of the self-advocates struggled to adapt, and supports that worked for paper timesheets were no longer helpful.

Through a careful engagement with the project takeaways, shared in a conversation by self-advocates during the final team meeting, it became evident who served on the team and how those people approached accessibility and team relationships deeply impacted how inclusive the project felt for self-advocates. One self-advocate shared that 'Who serves as self-advocate support matters.' As a part of this conversation, another self-advocate team member shared: 'Self-advocate support needs to not silence self-advocates.' Some of the people who were self-advocate support would ignore commentary from self-advocates and/or centre the conversation for the working group time on topics of interest to them or what they felt should be discussed. This happened both with support workers who came with the self-advocates, but also with people we hired to be part of the team to support the self-advocates. This even affected our efforts at accessibility when support people focused on their own personal accessibility needs. For example, one member of the self-advocate support team often talked about accessibility as connected to their own vision needs, as opposed to accessibility as explained/needed by self-advocates with intellectual disability. Self-advocates on the team specifically identified the importance of hiring self-advocate support who have experience working with people who self-identify as intellectually disabled. Self-advocates noted that: 'Accessibility for people with intellectual disability is very different from physical disabilities, vision disabilities, etc. [...] [self advocates] need an understanding of this population and knowledge about how to best draw on their strengths and capture their knowledge.'

Conclusion

Beyond the principles and challenges of PAR identified by Balcazar et al. (1998), members of the C4A team learned several important lessons. Yogi Berra is famously (and possibly apocryphally) quoted as saying: 'In theory there is no difference between theory and practice; in practice there is.' This quote is fitting because we found ourselves having to rethink our assumptions about many aspects of the project along the way. We learned that a commitment to a person-centred, participatory and inclusive design and development process requires a radically different approach than technology development processes that do not try to include people with intellectual disability. While this might seem an obvious observation (in theory), figuring out the different approaches would be was harder than we planned (also in theory) as there were few models or examples to draw on (in practice) because of the dearth of people with intellectual disability in the technology development world. If we were doing the work in the project over again, one thing we would probably do differently is have far fewer people on the team (at times the team numbered 20+ people) and have the entire group work on one tool rather than having multiple groups working simultaneously. We would plan to spend more time planning and build that into the overall project timeline and deliverables because the team spent more time on project management than would be the case with a less participatory team. The team's decision-making process was slower than if it were top-down only; moreover, it is important to document decisions in ways that are relevant and accessible to the entire team (i.e., the group cannot rely solely on written documentation and email threads to communicate). We would have focused on capacity building early on and before starting content development. A participatory development project by and for people with intellectual disability is hugely different from a project where 'experts' (in our case, academics) create specifications, hire developers and build some technology. When the project began, the team believed it would have depth in content areas (both team members with and without intellectual disability). From the start, the C4A project team included members with intellectual disability who had experience in self-advocacy. As the project unfolded, it proved more challenging to find people with intellectual disability with experience in any form of technology development. To address that issue, the team decided to recruit several members of the team who were very interested in technology and then work with them to build the knowledge and skills the project requires; however, it would have been better to build this capacity initially.

This chapter has offered some of the opportunities and challenges of using PAR in technology research and development. PAR can play an important role in the development of technology solutions for people with intellectual disabilities. By involving individuals with intellectual disability in the research process, PAR can ensure that the technology developed is both accessible and useful for its intended users. Moreover, PAR can empower individuals with intellectual disability to take an active role in the development of technology solutions that are designed to meet their unique needs. By involving them in the research process, PAR can provide opportunities for them to share their experiences and insights, and to co-create technology solutions that are tailored to their specific requirements.

PAR can also help challenge the assumptions and biases that often underpin both academic research and the development of technology for people with disabilities. PAR has the potential to increase self-esteem, self-efficacy and empowerment of a community that has historically been exploited and oppressed by research methods. PAR can also build capacity in the disability community and transform the relationships between the community and professional researchers. PAR also presents challenges, including the need to devote time to building relationships, create and provide accommodations to participate, and devise ways to share power over the nature and direction of research.

The future of PAR and technology development with people with intellectual disability is promising, as it has the potential to promote inclusion and empower individuals with intellectual disability to become more engaged and active members of their communities. However, there are also challenges and barriers that need to be addressed to ensure the success of PAR with people with intellectual disabilities. There is a continuing need for increased resources and support for individuals with intellectual disabilities to participate fully in PAR activities. This includes access to appropriate communication and assistive technologies, as well as training and support for PAR facilitators and researchers. Stigma and discrimination against people with intellectual disability can present a significant barrier to their participation in PAR activities. It is important to address these discriminatory and ableist attitudes to promote greater understanding and acceptance of individuals with intellectual disability.

Having a commitment to participant involvement throughout the process might make a project take longer, but the inclusion of people with intellectual disability must be more than just performative. In addition to helping ensure the appropriateness and usefulness of the technology being researched or developed, a participatory approach provides a team more opportunities for unexpected discoveries, chances to learn from each other and ideas for future work together.

Note

1.   https://sanys.org/who-we-are/mission/.

References

Amiel, T., & Reeves, T.C. (2008). Design-based research and educational technology: Rethinking technology and the research agenda. *Educational Technology & Society*, *11*(4), 29–40. https://www.j-ets.net/collection/published-issues/11_4

Balcazar, F., Keys, C., & Kaplan, D. (1998). Participatory action research and people with disabilities: Principles and challenges. *Canadian Journal of Rehabilitation*, *12*(2), 105–112.

Barton, L. (2005). Emancipatory research and disabled people: Some observations and questions. *Educational Review*, *57*(3), 317–327. https:// doi .org/ 10 .1080/ 00131910500149325

Beighton, C., Victor, C., Carey, I.M., Hosking, F., DeWilde, S., Cook, D.G., Manners, P., & Harris, T. (2019). 'I'm sure we made it a better study…': Experiences of adults with intellectual disabilities and parent carers of patient and public involvement in a health research study. *Journal of Intellectual Disabilities*, *23*(1), 78–96. https://doi .org/10.1177/1744629517723485

Bigby, C., & Frawley, P. (2010). Reflections on doing inclusive research in the 'Making Life Good in the Community' study. *Journal of Intellectual & Developmental Disability*, *35*(2), 53–61. https://doi.org/10.3109/13668251003716425

Broderick, A., & Lalvani, P. (2017). Dysconscious ableism: Toward a liberatory praxis in teacher education. *International Journal of Inclusive Education*, *21*(9), 894–905. https://doi.org/10.1080/13603116.2017.1296034

Cobb, P., Confrey, J., DiSessa, A., Lehrer, R., & Schauble, L. (2003). Design experiments in educational research. *Educational Researcher*, *32*(1), 9–13. https:// doi .org/ 10 .3102/0013189X032001009

Conder, J., Milner, P., & Mirfin-Veitch, B. (2011). Reflections on a participatory project: The rewards and challenges for the lead researchers. *Journal of Intellectual and Developmental Disability*, *36*(1), 39–48. https://doi.org/10.3109/13668250.2010 .548753

Davies, D.K., Stock, S.E., King, L.R., Brown, R.B., Wehmeyer, M.L., & Shogren, K.A. (2015). An interface to support independent use of Facebook by people with intellectual disability. *Intellectual and Developmental Disabilities*, *53*(1), 30–41. https://meridian.allenpress.com/idd/article-abstract/53/1/30/1639/An-Interface-to -Support-Independent-Use-of?redirectedFrom=fulltext

Dolmage, J. (2017). *Academic Ableism*. University of Michigan Press. https://doi.org/ 10.3998/mpub.9708722

Foley, A. (2019). Starting the process: Developing digital tools with and for people with intellectual disability. In D.L. Edyburn (Ed.), *App Development for Individuals with Disabilities: Insights for Developers and Entrepreneurs* (pp. 1–25). Knowledge by Design Inc.

Foley, A., & Ferri, B.A. (2012). Technology for people, not disabilities: Ensuring access and inclusion. *Journal of Research in Special Educational Needs, 12*(4), 192–200. https://doi.org/10.1111/j.1471-3802.2011.01230.x

Friedman, M., & Bryen, D.N. (2007). Web accessibility for people with cognitive disabilities. *Technology and Disability, 19,* 205–212. https://doi.org/10.1145/1056808.1057024

Guillaume, L. (2011). Critical race and disability framework: A new paradigm for understanding discrimination against people from non-English speaking backgrounds and Indigenous people with disability. *Critical Race and Whiteness Studies, 7,* 6–19.

Hammel, J., McDonald, K.E., & Frieden, L. (2016). Getting to inclusion: People with developmental disabilities and the Americans With Disabilities Act Participatory Action Research Consortium. *Inclusion, 4*(1), 6–15. https:// meridian .allenpress .com/ inclusion/ article -abstract/ 4/ 1/ 6/ 325/ Getting -to -Inclusion -People -With -Developmental

Harbour, W.S., & Greenberg, D. (2017). *Campus Climate and Students with Disabilities.* NCCSD Research Brief (Vol. 1, Issue 2). National Center for College Students with Disabilities.

Hynan, A., Goldbart, J., & Murray, J. (2015). A grounded theory of Internet and social media use by young people who use augmentative and alternative communication (AAC). *Disability and Rehabilitation, 37*(17), 1559–1575. https://doi.org/10.3109/09638288.2015.1056387

Knox, M., Mok, M., & Parmenter, T.R. (2000). Working with the experts: Collaborative research with people with an intellectual disability. *Disability & Society, 15*(1), 49–61. https://doi.org/10.1080/09687590025766

Larson, S., Salmi, P., Smith, D., Anderson, L., & Hewitt, A. (2013). *Residential services for persons with intellectual or developmental disabilities: Status and trends through 2011.* National Residential Information Systems Project (RISP), Research and Training Center on Community Living, Institute on Community Integration/ UCEDD, University of Minnesota.

McDonald, K.E., & Stack, E. (2016). You say you want a revolution: An empirical study of community-based participatory research with people with developmental disabilities. *Disability and Health Journal, 9*(2), 201–207. https://doi.org/10.1016/j.dhjo.2015.12.006

Miller, R.W. (2019). 'A gut punch': How the college admissions scandal hurt families with disabled students. *USA Today,* 16 March. https:// www .usatoday .com/ story/ news/education/2019/03/16/college-admissions-scandal-how-disabled-students-sat -act-test-accommodations/3164324002/

Minkler, M., Hammel, J., Gill, C., & Magasi, S. (2008). Community-based participatory research in disability and long-term care policy: A case study. *Journal of Disability Policy, 19*(2), 114–126.

Nicolaidis, C., Raymaker, D.M., Ashkenazy, E., McDonald, K.E., Dern, S., Baggs, A.E., Kapp, S.K., Weiner, M., & Boisclair, W.C. (2015). 'Respect the way I need to communicate with you': Healthcare experiences of adults on the autism spectrum. *Autism, 19*(7), 824–831. https://doi.org/10.1177/1362361315576221

Nicolaidis, C., Raymaker, D., McDonald, K., Dern, S., Ashkenazy, E., Boisclair, C., Robertson, S., & Baggs, A. (2011). Collaboration strategies in nontraditional community-based participatory research partnerships: Lessons from an academic–community partnership with autistic self-advocates. *Progress in Community Health Partnerships: Research, Education, and Action*, 5(2), 143–150. https:// doi .org/ 10 .1353/cpr.2011.0022

Nind, M., Chapman, R., Seale, J., & Tilley, L. (2016). The conundrum of training and capacity building for people with learning disabilities doing research. *Journal of Applied Research in Intellectual Disabilities*, 29(6), 542–551. https://doi.org/10.1111/jar.12213

Oden, K., Hernandez, B., & Hidalgo, M.A. (2010). Payoffs of participatory action research: Racial and ethnic minorities with disabilities reflect on their research experiences. *Community Development*, 41(1), 21–31. https:// doi .org/ 10 .1080/ 155 75330903477275

Sachdeva, N., Tuikka, A.-M., Kristian, K., & Reima Suomi, K. (2015). Digital disability divide in information society: A framework based on a structured literature review. *Journal of Information, Communication and Ethics in Society*, 13(3), 283–298. https://doi.org/10.1108/JICES-10-2014-0050

Shpigelman, C-N., & Gill, C.J. (2014). How do adults with intellectual disabilities use Facebook? *Disability & Society*, 29(10), 1601–1616. https:// doi .org/ 10 .1080/ 09687599.2014.966186

Sitbon, L. (2018). Engaging IT students in co-design with people with intellectual disability. *Extended Abstracts of the 2018 CHI Conference on Human Factors in Computing Systems*, 1–6. https://doi.org/10.1145/3170427.3188620

Sitbon, L., & Farhin, S. (2017). Co-designing interactive applications with adults with intellectual disability: A case study. *Proceedings of the 29th Australian Conference on Computer-Human Interaction*, 487–491. https://doi.org/10.1145/3152771.3156163

Stack, E., & McDonald, K.E. (2014). Nothing about us without us: Does action research in developmental disabilities research measure up? *Journal of Policy and Practice in Intellectual Disabilities*, 11(2), 83–91. https://doi.org/10.1111/jppi.12074

Vicente, M.R., & López, A.J. (2010). A multidimensional analysis of the disability digital divide: Some evidence for internet use. *The Information Society*, 26(1), 48–64. https://doi.org/10.1080/01615440903423245

Walker, D. (2006). Towards Productive Design Studies. In J. van den Akker, K. Gravemeijer, S. McKenney, & N. Nieveen (Eds.), *Educational Design Research* (pp. 8–14). Routledge.

Zhang, S., & Dorn, B. (2013). A community-based participatory research model and web application for studying health professional shortage areas in the United States. *International Journal of Healthcare Information Systems and Informatics*, 8(3), 23–37. https://doi.org/10.4018/jhisi.2013070102

4. Improving quality of life through the application of assistive technology

Paul Whittington and Huseyin Dogan

Introduction

The World Bank (n.d.) states that there are one billion people worldwide that have disabilities affecting daily interactions with society, which accounts for 15 per cent of the population worldwide. People with disabilities include those who have physical and cognition conditions that can result in associated impairments, such as those affecting finger dexterity, speech and vision. This user group often relies on assistive technologies to improve their quality of life and this is a continuously evolving domain. Quality of life is defined as "an individual's perception of their position in life in the context of the culture and value systems in which they live and in relation to their goals, expectations, standards and concerns" (World Health Organization, 2012). The use of assistive technology can allow increased independence and less reliance on others, therefore resulting in an improved quality of life. A common language for defining disability is the International Classification for Disability, Functioning and Health (ICF) developed by the World Health Organization (2001) and this is seen as the worldwide standard for disability classification. The aim of the ICF is to ensure that disability is considered as a "complex interaction between the person and the environment", rather than characterising individuals (Kostanjsek, 2011, p. 4).

This chapter is based on previous assistive technology research that developed the SmartAbility Framework to provide recommendations for assistive technologies based on users' physical abilities, i.e., actions performed independently. These recommendations are provided by an Android application connected to a database to retrieve specific assistive technologies that are suitable to the user's abilities. The SmartAbility Framework consists of five elements that are mapped together to consider the relationships between physical conditions, abilities, interaction mediums and assistive technologies.

This framework concept was established and evolved during four years of PhD research (Whittington & Dogan, 2016) and enhanced through three years of postdoctoral research (Whittington et al., 2018). During this period, four controlled usability evaluations were conducted, as well as two framework validations. This culminated in the involvement of approximately 100 participants, including those with reduced physical and cognitive abilities and domain experts with assistive technology, human-computer interaction and healthcare backgrounds.

Three assistive technology case studies are described in this chapter: Authentibility Pass, HealthAbility and EduAbility. Authentibility Pass is a proof-of-concept Android application that allows users with reduced abilities to communicate their authentication and accessibility requirements to organisations so that they can be authenticated in an accessible method. This has formed the basis of the HealthAbility concept, a customised version of Authentibility Pass in the healthcare domain, to provide a method for patients with disabilities to communicate their accessibility needs to healthcare professionals. EduAbility is a separate Android application, designed for the education domain, which provides assistive technology recommendations and training for teachers, support staff, parents and carers. This chapter will also discuss related work for each case study, the conducted usability evaluations, lessons learnt and the future directions. The aim is to provide an insight into the key findings from the research and the important considerations for future research in assistive technology.

Case study 1: Authentibility Pass

It has been identified that people with reduced abilities encounter barriers due to web security and privacy technologies. These challenges can include users with cognitive conditions experiencing difficulties following multi-step procedures on websites (World Wide Web Consortium, n.d.). Also, people with reduced abilities such as visual impairments, dyslexia and motor difficulties can experience challenges using authentication methods such as Personal Identification Number (PIN) codes, textual passwords and one-time codes received through Short Message Service (SMS) (Hayes et al., 2017; Helkala, 2012). Biometrics such as fingerprint and face detection are alternative authentication mechanisms that could be more suitable to certain disabilities, but this can raise privacy concerns (Blanco-Gonzala et al., 2018). Authentication mechanisms should be accessible to users of all physical and learning abilities, but these users often have to compromise on either security or usability

(Furnell et al., 2022). We identified that currently there is not a solution for communicating both authentication and accessibility requirements to organisations. This was the rationale behind developing Authentibility Pass, where users would only need to enter their requirements once into an application and communicate these to multiple organisations. This would be significantly less time-consuming than informing organisations separately.

Authentibility Pass enables people with physical and/or learning disabilities to communicate their authentication and accessibility requirements to organisations, such as financial institutions, small and medium-sized enterprises (SMEs), non-profit organisations, higher-education institutions and schools. The first stage of the development was to conduct a market validation to identify the current processes of communicating requirements within these organisations and their challenges, as well as gauging potential interest in a smartphone solution. Authentibility Pass comprises of an Android application, database, web interface and Application Programming Interface (API). We conducted our market validation by approaching representatives from each of the sectors, and the key findings are summarised here.

Financial institutions: Customers currently state their accessibility preferences, which are tagged to a customer profile by a frontline member of staff. However, one limitation is that the requirements are selected from a multiple-choice list, which may not accurately reflect a customer's needs. It was also highlighted that occasionally inconsistencies were generated when customer requirements were communicated across departments in large financial institutions. This domain would only consider integrating Authentibility Pass if it was able to interface with existing customer databases through an API.

SMEs: An organisation that frequently organises events has to currently obtain registration of delegates' accessibility and dietary requirements through an event management provider. One limitation is that the SMEs organising these events will only store this information while the event is taking place and then delete it. SMEs stated that Authentibility Pass would be beneficial in enabling customers to share and retain their accessibility requirements in advance, allowing more efficient planning of events.

Non-profit organisations: Authentibility Pass would be a valuable solution for 'Front of House' teams and Duty Managers, but it would need to be compatible with existing event management systems. Accessibility requirements for their customers are currently stored during the registration process for events, and the onus is therefore on customers to advise organisations of their requirements in advance. It was seen that the Authentibility application would be a more efficient solution to communicate and store visitor requirements.

Higher education: Authentibility Pass would be beneficial to students with a range of reduced abilities. Learning Support departments currently update a student record system with information on conditions, exam adjustments, Disabled Students' Allowance requirements and personal contact details. Authentibility Pass would provide the benefit of the database being accessible to all university staff, ensuring awareness of specific requirements of students, in order to provide efficient and holistic support.

User community: The market validation involved people with disabilities who highlighted the frequent challenges with communicating their authentication and accessibility requirements to organisations. They often need to repeatedly inform individual organisations of their requirements when attending events, and this can be difficult due to their reduced physical abilities.

Based on the findings from the market validation, a requirement specification was produced for Authentibility Pass, stating the functionality of the Android application, database, web interface and API. Volere Requirement Shells (Robertson & Robertson, 2009) were utilised to produce functional and non-functional requirements, which were categorised using Volere, including Security and Usability, and prioritised using MoSCoW (Clegg & Barker, 1994). This approach defined the 'Must Have', 'Should Have', 'Could Have' and 'Won't Have' requirements. 'Must Have' are the Minimum Usable SubseT (MUST) of requirements which a system guarantees to deliver, whereas 'Should Have' requirements are important but not vital. There are five key requirements and rationales for Authentibility Pass:

1. It shall be possible to search for customer authentication/accessibility requirements through the web interface. (Must Have)
2. The organisational database shall store a unique customer ID number, Authentibility Pass account details and customer authentication/accessibility requirements. (Must Have)
3. Token-based authentication shall be used to authenticate the user. (Must Have)
4. The application shall check whether users can operate specific verification techniques on a smartphone. (Should Have)
5. The verification check shall contain adequate instructions on each interface on how users should complete each check. (Should Have)

User Interface

The Authentibility Pass user interface is designed for people with disabilities to enter their authentication and accessibility requirements, which are stored in their account. Accessibility requirements include disability types, impairments and specific needs, for example if they are a United Kingdom (UK) Blue Badge holder,[1] which can be selected through checkboxes, as shown in Figure 4.1.

In the Authentication Requirements section (see Figure 4.2), users can state their authentication preferences in terms of the formats to receive one-time codes, as well as their abilities to remember passwords and PINs. The application will then ascertain the authentication methods compatible with a user's device to verify each of the available methods. A series of short checks will also be conducted to ascertain whether the user can operate each authentication method. If the user is unable to complete the check, the relevant authentication method will automatically be deselected from their requirements. Both the authentication and accessibility requirements will be stored in the user's Authentibility Pass account. Users will be able to select from a list which organisations they choose to send their accessibility and authentication requirements. Prior to sending their requirements, the user will need to be identified by the organisation, e.g., an account number or customer reference number.

Requirements are transmitted from the smartphone to the organisation database, using token-based authentication that encrypts data, so that the organisation with the correct token can decrypt the data. The web interface is designed for organisations to access customer requirements, enabling searches to be performed for requirements based on the customer ID or name. The web interface is specific for a particular organisation, allowing all of their customer requirements to be viewed. Organisation details can also be updated through the web interface and employees can then view the specific requirements of customers, in order to determine the most suitable method of interaction.

The private Authentibility Pass API is to be used by organisations that have existing database systems, and once registered they will be provided with a unique API key to facilitate integration with their existing database systems. The key is not publicly available, maintaining the integrity of Authentibility Pass. The API receives requirements sent from the Authentibility Pass application and transmits these to an organisation's database system in a range of supported file formats, e.g., Comma Separated Variables (CSV) files, where they are stored with the existing customer records.

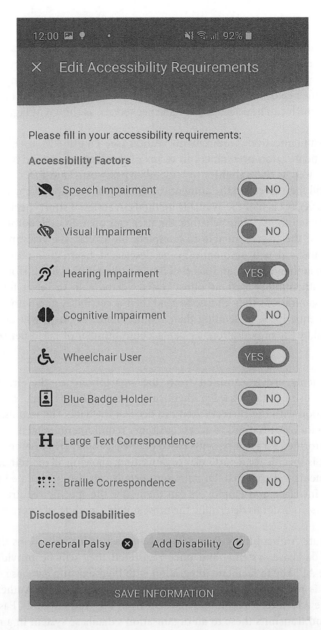

Figure 4.1   Input of accessibility requirements through the Android application

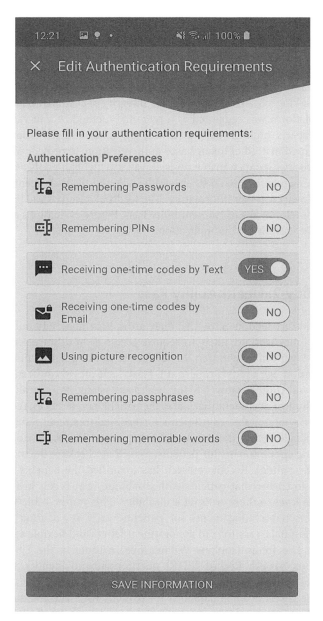

Figure 4.2   Input of authentication requirements through the Android application

Preliminary Evaluations

Authentibility Pass was presented to experts in the domains of cyber security and finance. The user interface received positive feedback from financial institutions who emphasised the importance of considering customers' accessibility needs. However, it would be essential for the application to integrate into the existing banking systems to maintain the integrity of customer data. The open banking platform was suggested as a potential method of integration. Cyber security experts highlighted that a cryptographic authentication protocol should be used instead of token-based authentication, to provide an increased level of security for data transmissions. It was also highlighted that Global Data Protection Regulations (GDPR) should be adhered to, as Authentibility Pass stores personal customer information. The feedback received will be addressed in future developments of Authentibility Pass. Future evaluations are planned to assess the usability of the application.

Case study 2: HealthAbility Pass

In the healthcare section of the UK, there are approximately 14 million people with disabilities who are likely to require access to healthcare services. This comprises 9 per cent of children, 21 per cent of working-age adults and 42 per cent of pension-age adults (Scope, n.d.). Trials have previously been conducted in the UK and United States (US) for 'healthcare passports'. A healthcare passport is a physical document that states the patient's preferences, requirements and necessary reasonable adjustments for hospital treatment. The purpose is to have a single record that the healthcare professional is able to view prior to arranging appointments for patients, as well as checking the record before meeting the patient. Recent research has identified the benefits of hospital passports, to ensure that patients with disabilities can access health services at an equal level to those without a disability. This can be achieved through making reasonable adjustments for patients, such as ensuring wheelchair access to hospitals, easy to read appointment letters and flexible appointment durations. The Johns Hopkins Wilmer Eye Institute in the US developed an Electronic Health Record (EHR) questionnaire to identify accessibility requests for patients at an eye clinic (Varadaraj et al., 2022). There have been trials in the UK of hospital passports for patients with learning disabilities to support communicating their needs to carers and hospital staff (Bell, 2012). In this trial, a Traffic Light Hospital Assessment Tool was developed for patients with learning disabilities in the form of an A4-size coloured booklet with red, amber and green sections to provide a patient with specific information. It was found that the tool was helpful in communicating patient requirements to clinicians, but there were challenges related to the tool not being recognised throughout some hospital departments. Additionally, Public Health England developed a Regional Hospital Passport for Individuals with Learning Disabilities (RHPLD), to provide information to assist hospital staff in considering reasonable adjustments for patient care (Millman & Gamble, 2018). Some NHS Trusts in the UK are currently implementing hospital passports, including Western Sussex NHS Foundation Trust, who utilise a My Care Passport (Western Sussex NHS Foundation Trust, n.d.) that contains information about patients and their needs on a paper-based document. Charities such as the Royal MENCAP Society also provide hospital passports, and there is evidence that these can save patients' lives (Mencap, n.d.).

HealthAbility Pass is a case study that is based on Authentibility Pass, where the existing Android application would be customised for the healthcare domain. Our research is at a conceptual stage, where the initial designs have been co-produced with healthcare experts from the University Hospitals Dorset National Health Service (NHS) Foundation Trust, Dorset Council and Dorset Healthcare University NHS Foundation Trust in the UK (Whittington et al., 2022). It is anticipated that this would be an innovative solution for patients to communicate their accessibility requirements to the desired clinicians and hospital staff, through token-based authentication. The aim of HealthAbility Pass would be for healthcare professionals to receive the requirements of patients in advance of their visit, so that they can be best supported on their arrival. The solution would have the following key features:

1. Patients only need to enter their requirements once, which can be sent to multiple hospitals.
2. Patients are in control of their own data, deciding which hospitals have access.
3. Hospitals are provided with a record of patients' accessibility requirements.
4. Hospitals with existing databases can use an API to receive requirements that are sent via the HealthAbility Pass application.

Preliminary Designs

Five one-hour co-creation meetings were held with the Accessibility Task Force at the Royal Bournemouth Hospital over nine months, to develop the HealthAbility Pass concept. Minutes were taken at each meeting and a total of 21 pages and 5,724 words were recorded. Based on these discussions, it was agreed that HealthAbility Pass would expand the accessibility requirements section of Authentibility Pass to include additional information required for hospital appointments. Initially, the focus would be on outpatient services, such as patients receiving treatment or having X-rays and computed tomography (CT) scans. The information would be used by clinicians ahead of a patient's appointment, so that the necessary arrangements can be made in advance.

Based on the initial feedback from the Accessibility Task Force on Authentibility Pass, the accessibility requirements would need to be expanded to allow users to also communicate their gender identity, cultural practices, transport and hoist requirements. As the range of accessibility requirements for patients is wide, it has been decided to separate these into domains and sub-domains, where each sub-domain will have a text field for patients to describe their specific requirements. The domains are aligned to the ICF with the first domain being 'Communication and Interaction', allowing patients to describe their condition in terms of speech impairments, dyslexia and autistic spectrum conditions. The next domain would consider 'Cognition and Learning' relating to learning disabilities or reading and writing challenges. The physical conditions of a patient would be considered in HealthAbility Pass within the 'Sensory and Physical' section of the application. This would include sensory impairments, physical disabilities and whether the patient is a wheelchair user or requires large text and Braille correspondence. Another section of patient requirements relating to 'Social, Emotional and Mental Health' would allow users to state a range of conditions, such as anxiety, depression and claustrophobia. The final section of the accessibility requirements would consider other aspects, such as the need for a personal assistant, dietary preferences or whether the patient is a UK Blue Badge holder.

A user-centred design approach would be adopted to develop HealthAbility Pass, which is an iterative process that focuses on the understanding of users and their context in all stages of design and development (Interaction Design Foundation, n.d.). Throughout this process the development would be conducted in collaboration with clinicians at University Hospitals Dorset and Dorset HealthCare University NHS Foundation Trust. Discussions would also be held with the Information Technology Departments of each of the Hospital Trusts, to determine the process of integrating HealthAbility Pass into their current systems. An initial requirements specification has been produced using Volere Requirements Shells. This is an internationally recognised technique developed by The Atlantic Systems Guild Ltd. that is used to define atomic requirements. These are requirements that are "measurable, testable, traceable and detailed enough to define all aspects of a need without further breakdown" (Robertson & Robertson, 2009, p.1). MoSCoW is a prioritisation technique for requirements (Clegg & Barker, 1994), which defines them in terms of 'Must Have', 'Should Have', 'Could Have' and 'Won't Have'. 'Must Have' requirements are non-negotiable for a system, 'Should Have' requirements are essential but not vital, whereas 'Could Have' requirements are not essential to the core functionality. 'Won't Have' requirements are those that can be considered for future development. The example functional, maintainability and performance requirements for HealthAbility Pass include:

1. HealthAbility Pass shall check the connection to the HealthAbility Pass database on start-up. (Must Have)
2. The Hospital database shall only store the NHS number and their accessibility requirements. (Must Have)
3. The Inform Hospitals interface should contain a list of hospitals that support HealthAbility Pass. (Should Have)
4. Hospitals shall be added or removed from the HealthAbility Pass database through the web application. (Should Have)

HealthAbility Pass is anticipated to increase the satisfaction of patients with disabilities. Hospitals would be made aware of specific needs so that clinicians and staff are more prepared to support patients on their arrival. The application would be integrated into the existing hospital systems through collaborations with the IT Departments.

Case study 3: EduAbility

In education, assistive technologies can be adopted to, 'increase, maintain or improve the social capabilities of persons with disabilities' (ATIA, n.d.). It is important to consider accessibility and inclusion, to ensure that people with special educational needs have equal access to opportunities. Past research studies have highlighted there is limited online educational resources related to assistive technology for teachers and support staff who support pupils with disabilities (UNESCO, 2019). Research also indicates there are challenges with personalising online educational resources, so that they can better support pupils with disabilities. In a World Bank Working Paper, Mcclain-Nhlapo et al. (2019) highlight that inclusive education requires the provision of reasonable adjustments tailored to the individual needs of the pupil. However, pupils can encounter inaccessible school curricula materials and inflexible learning assessments. There is evidence that Virtual Learning Environments (VLEs) do not consider the needs of pupils with multiple disabilities, due to the interfaces not being adaptable. Potential solutions include developing ontology-based personalisation of educational resources for pupils with disabilities through web communities (Nganji & Brayshaw, 2017). Alternatively, artificial intelligence (AI) can be used to customise Open Educational Resources (OER) and Massive Open Online Courses (MOOCs) to suit their accessibility needs (Shopland et al., 2022).

The EduAbility case study consists of an Android application developed to consider assistive technology for education and how products can be recommended to pupils who have special educational needs and disabilities. EduAbility is designed for people with reduced physical and cognitive abilities, teachers, support staff and parents or carers. The application builds on our SmartAbility Framework (Whittington et al., 2018) by supplementing the physical abilities with cognitive abilities stated in the World Health Organization's ICF Checklist (World Health Organization, 2003). EduAbility aligns with the UK Government's strategy 'Realising the potential of technology in education' that promotes the use of education assistive technologies within schools.

User Interface Design

The EduAbility application contains an assistive technology recommendation system and a training package. The recommendation system was developed based on the SmartAbility Framework and maps assistive technology products to the pupil's physical and cognitive abilities. Abilities can be entered into the application using a traffic light style grading system of 'Easy', 'Difficult' or 'Impossible', as shown in Figure 4.3. The application then connects with a database of assistive technology products. The database was created during the development of EduAbility and contains 50 products, including hardware and software, which are mapped to the required abilities. Based on the user's abilities, assistive technology recommendations are provided containing product details and website links for further information.

EduAbility also includes a training package which delivers assistive technology training for teachers, teaching assistants and support staff in schools, to increase their knowledge and awareness. The application will promote inclusivity in schools for pupils with disabilities, by training staff in suitable assistive technologies that can provide support. The training package contains three sections: Training, Learn and Videos.

As shown in Figure 4.4, the Training section consists of information in relation to categories of assistive technology hardware and software. The information provided is based on data obtained through online sources and

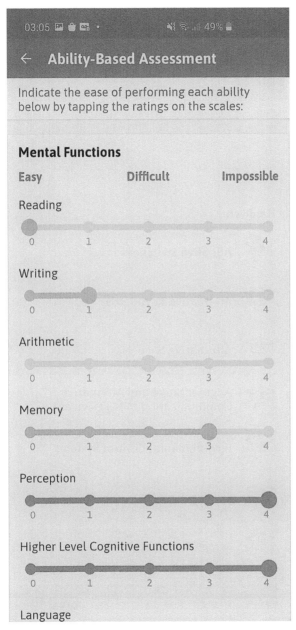

Figure 4.3   EduAbility recommendation system showing input of abilities

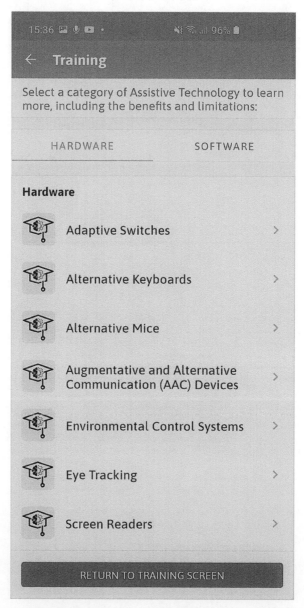

Figure 4.4   The EduAbility training package containing assistive technology hardware and software information

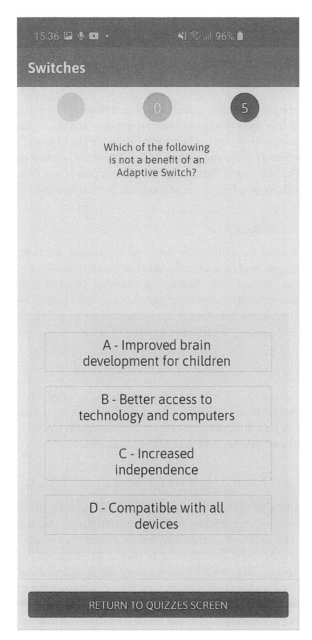

Figure 4.5   The EduAbility training package containing multiple-choice quizzes

describes the benefits and limitations of each type of product. Each category has a five-question multiple-choice quiz to test the user understanding of the various types of assistive technology (see Figure 4.5). Each quiz has a pass mark of 80 per cent, and the results are stored in the user's EduAbility profile to maintain a record of conducted training.

The Learn section contains online assistive technology articles, to provide users with further information on general applications of use for technology products. The application provides links to Portable Data Format (PDF) documents of academic papers and press releases. The Video section provides links to YouTube videos that illustrate real-world examples of assistive technology, to provide additional information and context on assistive technologies.

EduAbility Evaluation

The evaluations of the EduAbility Android application are being conducted with mainstream and special educational needs schools in Dorset and Hampshire, as well as with Additional Learning Support staff in Student Services at Bournemouth University. The purpose of the evaluation is to obtain initial feedback on the EduAbility application prior to public release. These evaluations will continue with future analysis of results.

Participants

Suitable schools were identified and contacted to arrange 30-minute video calls with representatives, including head teachers and support staff. A focus group was also held with academics from Bournemouth University who have expertise in the computing and accessibility domains.

Procedure

A demonstration of the application was provided and the participants were invited to download EduAbility on their Android device through the Google Play Store. The application was distributed through a Google Play Closed Test, where permissions were granted to invited participants. A 'think aloud' protocol (Nielsen, 2012) was followed, where the participants were provided with a usability evaluation pack containing instructions on interacting with the recommendation system and training package. Five tasks were then provided to participants; for example, 'To find suitable assistive technologies for a user with cerebral palsy'. The pack also contained two questionnaires, based on the System Usability Scale (SUS) (Brooke, 1996) and NASA Task Load Index (TLX) (NASA, n.d.). Using the SUS, participants rated ten statements on a five-point scale from 'Strongly Disagree' to 'Strongly Agree'. This allowed a single score to be calculated for the overall usability of EduAbility, which can be interpreted using the Adjective Rating Scale (Bangor et al., 2009) in terms of 'Poor', 'Good' or 'Excellent' usability. The NASA TLX provides measurements of Physical, Mental, Temporal, Performance, Effort and Frustration demands and can be implemented with a minimal amount of training, using either an iOS application developed by NASA or a paper-based version provided in the training package. The focus group was presented with a demonstration video of EduAbility and three trigger questions:

1. Which features of EduAbility do you prefer?
2. Can you identify any limitations on the functionality of EduAbility?
3. Can you suggest any improvements to EduAbility?

An open discussion was held with the focus group participants and feedback was collated. Initial evaluations have also been conducted with an Additional Learning Support department at a UK university. Participants evaluated the EduAbility application on an Android device. The findings from the focus group and initial evaluations suggested minor improvements to the user interface to improve screen navigation. The participants also acknowledged challenges of ensuring the product information in the database is maintained and updated. Positive feedback was also received in respect of the EduAbility application's benefits to students who are transitioning from schools to higher education and increasing their awareness of available assistive technologies to support their learning experience. This feedback and the findings from subsequent evaluations will be considered in future iterations of the development prior to public release. An iOS version will also be developed based on the consolidation Android application. Once both versions of EduAbility have been developed, they will initially be made freely available to the user community. This would be via digital distribution platforms or through websites of associations connected with disabilities. Depending on the popularity of the SmartAbility Application, a download fee could be introduced to support ongoing maintenance and updates to EduAbility. It is anticipated that EduAbility will develop into a product promotion tool for assistive technology manufacturers and charities, whereby their products can be promoted to the user community.

A future assistive technology research agenda

The three assistive technology case studies of Authentibility Pass, HealthAbility Pass and EduAbility will evolve through continued research conducted by Bournemouth University, to establish a research agenda that encompasses the education, financial and healthcare domains.

Potential organisations within the target market will be identified for Authentibility Pass, which have interactions with people who have physical and cognitive disabilities. The possibility of integrating the application with existing verification mechanisms and event management platforms will also be explored, such as the UK Government Gateway User ID, Eventbrite and Ticketmaster. Revenue streams will be established with different licensing packages, based on the type of organisation. Initially, free trials would be provided to organisations with limited functionality and a full version made available through an annual subscription. An iOS implementation of the application will be developed to increase the number of supporting organisations and users with reduced abilities. This will result in Authentibility Pass becoming a gateway for people with reduced abilities to communicate their authentication and accessibility requirements.

The HealthAbility Pass concept will evolve into a prototype application through continued collaboration with University Hospitals Dorset and Dorset HealthCare University NHS Foundation Trusts. This will result in Authentibility Pass being developed into a version that is suitable for healthcare to increase patient satisfaction. It will be essential to collaborate with the Hospital IT Department, to ensure HealthAbility Pass can be integrated within the existing hospital systems. The solution is anticipated to increase the satisfaction of patients with disabilities, as hospitals will be made aware of specific needs and clinicians and staff will be more prepared to support patients on their arrival. Once an application has been developed for the Dorset NHS Foundation Trusts, other Hospital Trusts will be approached for integration of HealthAbility Pass into their systems.

The Android and iOS EduAbility applications will be disseminated through mainstream and special educational needs schools, initially focusing on the region of Dorset and Hampshire, before considering a national launch. EduAbility will also be released as a freely available application to maximise interest and this could be converted into a paid version to support the longevity of the application. To provide international dissemination, the EduAbility applications will be translated into a variety of languages including Arabic and

Turkish, so that they have the potential to benefit people with reduced abilities worldwide. The usefulness of the recommendations provided by EduAbility will be measured in terms of abandonment rates of the suggested assistive technologies after specific timeframes, such as a week, month and year (Leckie, 2010). As an additional method of validation, the recommendations provided from EduAbility will be compared to those provided by human experts, such as occupational therapists. The results of these comparisons will ascertain the efficiency of EduAbility.

We have additional research initiatives to improve quality of life through assistive technology. This includes the development of a smart powerchair that will investigate integrating off-the-shelf technology into a powered wheelchair. The aim will be to increase the ability for the powerchair to support daily tasks for people who have mobility challenges. A potential area that will be explored is the autonomous navigation of the powerchair through image processing and light detection and ranging (LiDAR) technology, to provide a solution for transportation in vehicles. This will further develop our previous SmartATRS research (Whittington et al., 2015) based on the Automated Transport and Retrieval System (ATRS) (Gao et al., 2008).

Conclusions

Authentibility Pass, HealthAbility Pass and EduAbility are examples of how quality of life can be improved for people with disabilities through the application of assistive technology.

Authentibility Pass will improve the satisfaction of customers with reduced abilities, as organisations will become more aware of their authentication and accessibility requirements. This will be achieved through dissemination to higher educational institutions, schools, non-profit organisations, SMEs and financial institutions. This will result in Authentibility Pass becoming a gateway for people with reduced abilities to communicate their authentication and accessibility requirements. The application will be customised for healthcare in the form of HealthAbility Pass. This application will become an accessible healthcare gateway for patients with disabilities, to communicate their accessibility requirements to clinicians and hospital staff in advance of their visits.

The aim of EduAbility is to supplement the assistive technology assessments that are currently performed by domain experts, such as occupational therapists. The recommendations vary depending on a user's abilities, as there is not a 'single solution to fit multiple needs', similar to the 'One Size Fits All' Information Technology concept (Adams, 2017). However, one limitation of the EduAbility assessment is that an individual may prefer human interaction, or may not be able to use a smartphone. It is envisaged that the application could be used as an initial assessment tool, prior to visits to domain experts. This would be beneficial to reduce travelling time and costs, potentially enabling a greater number of assessments to be performed. A manual assessment could be subsequently arranged to obtain further information or for demonstrations of the recommended assistive technologies.

The common theme presented in each of our case studies is the application of assistive technology to a variety of real-world situations, to enhance and improve the quality of life for people with disabilities. Our research has shown that raising awareness of assistive technologies is essential to ensure that they can benefit this user community who can often be unaware of the products that are available. Therefore, assessments for people with disabilities and training for parents/carers, teachers and support staff should be the focus of the research agenda for the domain. It is also important to consider that there is never a single assistive technology solution that suits everyone, and recommendations should be customised for people's abilities. The field of assistive technology is continuously evolving and it is challenging to remain informed of the latest product developments. However, the provision of recommendations and training will help people with disabilities to benefit from the full potential of assistive technologies.

Note

1.   In the UK, local councils issue people with disabilities with a 'Blue Badge', which entitles them to park their vehicle closer to their destination.

References

Adams, J. (2017). *The High Cost of a One Size Fits All Technology Approach.* https://blogs.poly.com/high-cost-one-size-fits-technology-approach/
ATIA (n.d.). *What is AT?* Assistive Technology Industry Association. https://www.atia.org/at-resources/what-is-at/
Bangor, A., Kortrum, P., & Miller, J. (2009). Determining what individual SUS scores mean: Adding an adjective rating scale. *Usability Studies, 4*(3), 114–123. https://dl.acm.org/doi/10.5555/2835587.2835589

Bell, R. (2012). Does he have sugar in his tea? Communication between people with learning disabilities, their carers and hospital staff. *Tizard Learning Disability Review, 17*(2), 57–63. https://doi.org/10.1108/13595471211218712

Blanco-Gonzala, R., Lunerti, C., Sanchez-Reillo, R., & Guest, R.M. (2018). Biometrics: Accessibility challenge or opportunity? *PLoS ONE, 13*(3): e0194111. https://doi.org/10.1371/journal.pone.0194111

Brooke, J. (1996). SUS: A Quick and Dirty Usability Scale. In P.W. Jordan, B. Thomas, I.L. McClelland, & B. Weerdmeester (Eds.), *Usability Evaluation in Industry* (pp. 189–194). CRC Press.

Clegg, D., & Barker, R. (1994). *Case Method Fast-Track: A RAD Approach.* Addison-Wesley. https://dl.acm.org/doi/10.5555/561543

Furnell, S., Helkala, K., & Woods, N. (2022). Accessible authentication: Assessing the applicability for users with disabilities. *Computers & Security, 113* (February 2022), 102561. https://doi.org/10.1016/j.cose.2021.102561

Gao, C., Miller, T., Spletzer, J.R., Hoffman, I., & Panzarella, T. (2008). Autonomous docking of a smart wheelchair for the Automated Transport and Retrieval System (ATRS). *Journal of Field Robotics, 25*(4–5), 203–222. https://doi.org/10.1002/rob.20236

Hayes, J., Xi, L., & Yang, W. (2017). 'I always have to think about it first': Authentication experiences of people with cognitive impairments. *Proceedings of the 19th International ACM SIGACCESS Conference on Computers and Accessibility (ASSETS '17)* (pp. 357–358). Association for Computing Machinery. https://doi.org/10.1145/3132525.3134788

Helkala, K. (2012). Disabilities and authentication methods: Usability and security. *Proceedings of the Seventh International Conference on Availability, Reliability and Security* (pp. 327–334). DOI:10.1109/ARES.2012.19

Interaction Design Foundation (n.d.). *User Centered Design.* Interaction Design Foundation. https://www.interaction-design.org/literature/topics/user-centered-design

Kostanjsek, N. (2011). Use of the international classification of functioning, disability and health (ICF) as a conceptual framework and common language for disability statistics and health information systems. *Public Health, 11*(4), 1–6. https://doi.org/10.1186/1471-2458-11-S4-S3

Leckie, C. (2010). *The Abandonment of Technology.* Resilience. http://www.resilience.org/stories/2010-10-16/abandonment-technology/

Mcclain-Nhlapo, C.V., Cortez, C.J., Duchicela, L.F., & Lord, J.E. (2019). *Equity and Inclusion in Education in World Bank Projects: Persons with Disabilities, Indigenous Peoples, and Sexual and Gender Minorities.* The World Bank. http://documents1.worldbank.org/curated/en/590781562905434693/pdf/Equity-and-Inclusion-in-Education-in-World-Bank-Projects-Persons-with-Disabilities-Indigenous-Peoples-and-Sexual-and-Gender-Minorities.pdf

Mencap (n.d.). *Hospital Passports.* The Royal MENCAP Society. https://www.mencap.org.uk/advice-and-support/health-coronavirus/health-guides?fbclid=IwAR3OLetL_c2dl275FNry1nzJa_eG2hQ4Dj5T0wMWi84Nw27Daiekj1eEY0c

Millman, C., & Gamble, R. (2018). *Evaluation of the Regional Hospital Passport for People with Learning Disabilities.* Queen's University Belfast. https://niopa.qub.ac.uk/bitstream/NIOPA/11085/1/Evaluation%20of%20the%20RHPLD%20-%20Final%20publish.pdf

NASA (n.d.). *NASA TLX: Task Load Index.* National Aeronautics and Space Administration. https://humansystems.arc.nasa.gov/groups/tlx/

Nganji, J.T., & Brayshaw, M. (2017). Disability-aware adaptive and personalised learning for students with multiple disabilities. *International Journal of Information and Learning Technology, 34*(4), 307–321. https://doi.org/10.1108/IJILT-08-2016-0027

Nielsen, J. (2012). *Thinking Aloud: The #1 Usability Tool*. Nielsen Norman Group. https://www.nngroup.com/articles/thinking-aloud-the-1-usability-tool/

Robertson, R., & Robertson, S. (2009). *Atomic Requirements: Where the Rubber Hits the Road*. https://www.volere.org/wp-content/uploads/2018/12/06-Atomic-Requirements.pdf

Scope (n.d.). *Disability Facts and Figures*. Scope. https:// www .scope .org .uk/ media/ disability-facts-figures/

Shopland, N., Brown, D.J., Daniela, L., Rudolfa, A., Arifur, M., Rahman, A.B., Mahmud, M., & van Isacker, K. (2022). Improving Accessibility and Personalisation for HE Students with Disabilities in Two Countries in the Indian Subcontinent – Initial Findings. In M. Antona & C. Stephanidis (Eds.), *Universal Access in Human-Computer Interaction. User and Content Diversity. HCII 2022. Lecture Notes in Computer Science, vol 13309* (pp. 110–122). Springer. https://doi.org/10.1007/978 -3-031-05039-8_8

The World Bank (n.d.). *Disability Inclusion*. The World Bank. http://www.worldbank .org/en/topic/disability

UNESCO (2019). *Recommendation on Open Educational Resources (OER)*. United Nations Educational, Scientific and Cultural Organization. https://unesdoc.unesco .org/ark:/48223/pf0000373755/PDF/373755eng.pdf.multi.page=3

Varadaraj, V., Guo, X., & Reed, N.S. (2022). Identifying accessibility requests for patients with disabilities through an electronic health record-based questionnaire. *JAMA Network Open, 5*(4):e226555. https://doi.org/10.1001/jamanetworkopen.2022 .6555

Western Sussex NHS Foundation Trust (n.d.). *This is Me My Care Passport*. National Health Service. https://www.uhsussex.nhs.uk/resources/this-is-me-my-care-passport/

Whittington, P., Dogan, H., Phalp, K., & Phillips, J. (2022, 14–16 October). Health Ability Pass: An accessible healthcare gateway for patients with disabilities. *Proceedings of the IEEE International Conference on e-Business Engineering, ICEBE 2022* (pp. 282–287). DOI:10.1109/ICEBE55470.2022.00056

Whittington, P., Dogan, H., Jiang, N., & Phalp, K. (2018). Automatic detection of abilities through the SmartAbility framework. *Proceedings of the 32nd International BCS Human Computer Interaction Conference* (Article no. 43). ACM. https://doi.org/10 .14236/ewic/HCI2018.43

Whittington, P., & Dogan, H. (2016). A SmartDisability framework: Enhancing user interaction. *Proceedings of the 30th International BCS Human Computer Interaction Conference BCS HCI* 2016, pp. 1–11. BCS. DOI:10.14236/ewic/HCI2016.24

Whittington, P., Dogan, H., & Phalp, K. (2015). Evaluating the usability of an automated transport and retrieval system. *Proceedings of the International Conference on Pervasive and Embedded Computing and Communication Systems (PECCS 2015)* (pp. 49–66). IEEE. https://ieeexplore.ieee.org/document/7483733

World Health Organization (2012). *The World Health Organization Quality of Life (WHOQOL)*. World Health Organization. https://www.who.int/publications-detail -redirect/WHO-HIS-HSI-Rev.2012.03

World Health Organization (2003). *ICF Checklist*. World Health Organization. https:// www.who.int/publications/m/item/icf-checklist/

World Health Organization (2001). *International Classification of Functioning, Disability and Health (ICF) Framework*. The World Health Organization. https:// www .who .int/ standards/ classifications/ international -classification -of -functioning -disability-and-health

World Wide Web Consortium (n.d.). *Understanding Success Criterion 3.3.8: Accessible Authentication*. W3C. Retrieved 12 July 2023 from: https:// www .w3 .org/ WAI/ WCAG22/Understanding/accessible-authentication-minimum

5. An alternate approach to accessibility involving auto-hyper-personalisation

Gregg Vanderheiden, Crystal Marte and J. Bern Jordan

Introduction

Over the past 40 years, the field of information and communication technology (ICT) accessibility has seen significant progress. What started with 'special devices for special people' evolved into public and company-specific accessibility guidelines, international standards and accessibility laws worldwide. Many large companies have dedicated teams to improve accessibility and have built significant accessibility features directly into their products. The growing emphasis on accessibility in the industry has given rise to consultants, accessibility evaluation and remediation companies, and training programmes aimed at developing, training and certifying accessibility specialists.

Despite the progress made in accessibility, however, there are still major shortcomings. Audits of the field reveal that a low percentage of websites and products are accessible. Moreover, while some products have built-in accessibility features, they are only accessible to some individuals with disabilities. For example, smartphone screen readers with their gesture controls are fantastic for some blind users but are too complicated or physically impossible for others who are blind. Additionally, many/most products fail to effectively address the range of cognitive, language and learning disabilities, even though this is cumulatively the largest disability group.[1]

While we have made great progress from essentially zero products accessible to anyone 40 years ago, today there are still only a fraction of products that are accessible. Even the best among these are still inaccessible to a wide range of individuals. In sum:

- there are no products that are accessible across all of the different types, degrees and combinations of disability;

- there are a small number of products that are reasonably accessible across disabilities, but even those are only accessible to more typical or able individuals (e.g., those who are blind but are more digitally adroit versus the full range of people who are blind and who may have other disabilities).

While it is essential to continue moving forward with our traditional methods, there is also a need to consider augmenting them with new approaches that:

- can reach the large number of individuals who are currently left out; and
- require less effort so more companies are willing and able to make their products accessible.

Recent and emerging advances in technology may give us the tools to do this.

The evolution of ICT accessibility

The story of technology and disability began by creating 'special products for special people' – that is, people took mainstream technologies and developed special assistive technologies (ATs) for people with disabilities. In the 1960s, people used telephone stepper relays and typewriters with solenoids attached to their keys to create different types of sip-and-puff, scanning and other typewriters that allowed people who had very limited movement to communicate and write (Vanderheiden & Grilley, 1976; Copeland, 1974). With the advent of digital logic and then microprocessors, solid state communication and writing aids emerged. The first portable microprocessor-controlled aid, the Auto-Monitoring Communication Board (AutoCom), was released by the Trace Center in 1973 (Vanderheiden et al., 1973).

In 1978, Al Overby at IBM Raleigh developed a prototype system called SAID (Synthetic Audio Interface Driver). It was an IBM 3270 terminal connected to a 12-key telephone keypad and a Votrax synthesiser the size of a suitcase. SAID was later released as an IBM product called the Talking Terminal. Around this time, the IBM PC was released. Jim Thatcher and Jim Wright had newly joined IBM and had the idea to emulate SAID on the PC, which they called the PCSAID project, and make a much cheaper talking terminal, costing around $800 (1984).[2] These were the first known screen readers. Eventually, this became IBM Screen Reader for DOS, which was released in 1986 (see Keates, 2006).

Efforts at computer access began in earnest with the introduction of personal computers (Atari, TRS-80, Commodore, Apple, etc.) in the 1970s, which provided widely available, easily programmable computers. People began writing programs that would turn the microcomputer into dedicated ATs, e.g., programs to create a talking terminal (see earlier), a talking typewriter for people who are blind, a communication and writing aid for someone who is paralysed, etc.

Although initial devices were usually purpose-built for people with disabilities, it became quickly apparent that there was a need to move beyond special programs that turned computers into special devices for people with disabilities. Work then began on what was termed 'transparent access' (Vanderheiden, 1983). Transparent access refers to the ability of the disabled person to access the computer in such a way that the computer program cannot detect that the input is not coming to it in the standard fashion (from the standard keyboard and/or mouse). For example, if a program normally accepts input from the computer's keyboard, a transparent access technique would allow users to inject keystrokes (generated using sip-and-puff or scanning, etc.) in such a way that it is impossible for the program to tell that the input is not coming from the keyboard. With transparent access techniques, people with disabilities would be able to fully use the computer for all the same reasons and with all of the same software as everyone else.

An early example of this was the 'Dual Nested Computer Approach' proposed by Vanderheiden (1981) to address the fact that a lot of software directly accessed input hardware in the early days. One computer could act as a special interface (scanning, encoding, other) to a second computer – where the first was connected to the second through a keyboard-emulating interface (KEI), which made the output of the first computer look like it was a standard keyboard (and or mouse) to the second computer. As a result, the individuals could use the second computer to do all the same things that anyone else was able to do.

The most clever and innovative early approach to transparent access was the Adaptive Firmware Card (AFC) for the Apple IIe by Paul Schwejda. Because the Apple IIe had no operating system, software would directly read user keystrokes from the hardware keyboard encoder. As a result, it was not possible for ATs to inject themselves between the keyboard and the software as is done in modern operating systems. On the Apple IIe the keyboard encoder was memory mapped (i.e., it appeared as just an address in memory). Paul created a clever mechanism whereby the AFC would detect whenever the keyboard encoder address was read. When it detected that memory location being read, the AFC would do a 'system interrupt' and take control. The AFC program would then examine the program running at the time to see where the data were put that were read from the keyboard encoder. If it was null (i.e., there was no key pressed on the standard keyboard), the AFC would replace the null with whatever character the user had generated with the AFC's alternate input technique (e.g., scanning, encoding, sip-and-puff Morse code, etc.) and then return control to the computer. The computer program would come out of interrupt and process the (replaced) keystroke as if it had come from the keyboard (Schwejda & Vanderheiden, 1982). This was the first and earliest example of a single computer that, with the adapter firmware card, was able to provide transparent access to all the software running on the computer (the card also allowed users to slow down games to make them easier to play for people with disabilities and more).

Keyboard-emulating interfaces evolved into general input device-emulating interfaces that could simulate both keyboard and mouse and allow any augmentative communication aid to be used as an alternate keyboard and mouse for any computer. Standards were developed for this by the Trace Center – first the Keyboard Emulating Interface (KEI) Standard, and then the General Input Device Emulating Interface (GIDEI) standard (Schauer et al., 1994). GIDEI was later adopted in Access Pack for Windows (distributed by the Trace Center and Microsoft), AccessDOS (From IBM and Microsoft), and Serial Keys (found in AccessDOS, Windows95, ISO/IEC 9241–171, and an independent program called AAC Keys) (Vanderheiden et al., 2022).

With modern desktop operating systems (Windows, Mac OS, and Linux), it is now possible to run adaptive software, screen readers, alternate input methods, etc., on the same computer using multitasking and application programming interfaces (APIs) provided by the OS to inject keyboard and mouse events, so, except in special circumstances, hardware-based input-emulating interfaces are no longer needed. However, in mobile devices, the operating system (e.g., iOS and Android) sandboxes each app – preventing any app from affecting others. Although this security measure helps protect mobile devices from malware and other security threats, it prevents the use of third-party ATs. As a result, third-party ATs cannot be created for mobile systems in the same way they can for desktop operating systems. To address this problem, companies (Apple, Google, etc.) have started building a wide array of ATs directly into their mobile platforms to provide the functions normally provided by third-party ATs.[3] The benefit of this is that the ATs are free and built right into every product before it is shipped. The disadvantage is that if the particular type, degree or combination of disability that an individual has is not covered by the AT features on their mobile device, then there is no way for a third party to create an AT for that user/group.

Guidelines, Policies and Standards

Starting in 1985 a series of guidelines were developed to make ICTs accessible. The first were those created by the Trace Center (1985) on computer access for the White House (see Vanderheiden et al., 2022), followed by hardware and software accessibility guidelines developed by Trace for Apple for internal use (1986), with IBM for their internal use (1988) and for ITF foundation (1994) for consumer products (1990) and for Web content in 1995[4] and in 1997.[5] These were later picked up by Microsoft and other companies and used within their organisations and with their developers. Eventually, they were picked up and expanded in conjunction with others as part of broader efforts, including the W3C WCAG, Section 255, Section 508, HFES 200, ISO/IEC 9241–171 and 9241–151, EN 301 549, and other standards and regulatory documents (see Vanderheiden et al., 2022).

Currently there is a wide range of accessibility standards and regulations, with new ones being developed to address specific target technologies like self-service terminal machines (SSTMs), voting, etc. (Lazar et al., 2019). However, despite the range of guidelines and regulations, lawsuits to enforce them, and organisations devoted to helping companies create more accessible products or train accessibility professionals, most websites and products do not meet minimum accessibility standards and those that are considered accessible are not accessible to a large number of people with multiple disabilities and even for some single disabilities.

Where We Are

Today we are seeing a rapid proliferation of digital interfaces on everything from computers and mobile devices to stoves, thermostats, home security systems, hotel entertainment systems, drapes and thermostatic control and lighting of very modern hotel rooms, leaving people who need ATs in order to access these systems completely unable to operate them. Almost all of these are closed products that have very few or no accessibility features and there is no way to add any accessibility to these products – putting them out of reach of anybody who needs AT because they cannot use the standard interface.

In short, we have reached the point where operating digital interfaces is a requirement for getting an education and employment, daily living health-care, even operating your car – all things that 40 years ago, you were able to do without having to access a digital interface. If one cannot access these digital interfaces, one cannot live independently or even effectively in the world we are creating.

Coupling this with the low percentage of products that have accessibility and the essentially zero percentage of products that are available to individuals with all types, degrees and combinations of disability, it is clear that we need to have an alternate approach to fill the growing gap of products:

- that people need access to, but do not have accommodations for;
- that are closed and with which current ATs cannot be used;
- that are not accessible even with their built-in features to people with many types, degrees and combinations of disability.

Emerging technologies

A big question is whether emerging technologies will enable us to address the growing and existing problems described earlier. As a prelude to talking about this, it is helpful to briefly introduce some of the emerging technologies that we are seeing that can play a part in solving this problem.

Advancements in human–computer interaction are expanding at an unprecedented rate. With the current and future capabilities of artificial intelligence (AI), computer vision, brain–computer interfaces, sensors (and so on) – systems will go beyond direct commands to anticipate needs, customise interfaces and provide support in ways we are only beginning to imagine. The relationship between individuals and their digital and physical environments will become harmonious.

Computer-generated Text Will Be Human-indistinguishable from Human-generated Text for Most People

Although the technology behind the chatbot had been brewing behind the scenes in research labs and major tech companies for years, in November 2022, OpenAI released ChatGPT, which quickly became the fastest-expanding consumer software application in history – with over 100 million users by January 2023.[6] With this exponential growth, large technology corporations like Google, Baidu and Meta responded by accelerating the development of their competing products, such as Bard, Ernie Bot and LLaMA. Additionally, GPT-4, the large language model (LLM), has been integrated into Be My Eyes, a platform aiding visually impaired individuals in identifying objects and navigating their surroundings more effectively.[7]

Today, computer-generated text that uses LLMs and generative AI is nearly indistinguishable from human-generated text. For example, in a recent study conducted by researchers at the Institute of Biomedical Ethics and History of Medicine in Switzerland, participants found it difficult to discern between AI-generated (using GPT-3) and human writing. Interestingly, the researchers found that disinformation generated by AI was more believable to participants than what was written by humans (Spitale et al., 2023). In the future, the assumption is that this will be completely indistinguishable for most people and will be better and more accurate than that created by most people.

Computer-generated Speech Will Be Human-indistinguishable from Human Speech for Most People

Computer-generated speech (CGS) is now being used in a variety of applications, including virtual assistants (e.g., Siri, Alexa, Google Assistant), educational software, media production and customer service. Recently, there have been significant advances in the ability of computers to generate speech that is both intelligible and natural sounding. For example, Google's AudioLM is an audio generation framework that can create speech that continues in the accent and cadence of the original speaker (Borsos et al., 2023).

As machine learning techniques continue to improve, CGS models will become even more capable of generating speech that is indistinguishable from human speech and has significant improvements in naturalness, context awareness and variety. These advancements will open up new possibilities for CGS applications in various fields, including education, healthcare and entertainment.

Linguistic Transformations Will Be Seamless, Including Things that Require Semantic Understanding

A linguistic transformation refers to altering or changing the structure, form or content of language, often to convey the same information in a different way. Preliminary evidence shows that LLMs can simplify intricate text and adjust the reading level to match a user's needs.[8] However, there are still high error bars and issues with accuracy, and oversimplifying the text too much can cause it to lose its intended meaning.

In the future, simplifying complex text or language will be easier and more accurate. Going beyond reading levels, we will also be able to quickly translate text into different languages, whether it is Simplified English or another language. This capability would allow the separation of content creation from accessibility concerns – in other words, content could be made accessible to everyone, no matter its original form and no matter the language abilities of any individual.

Bidirectional Production and Recognition of ASL Will Be Significantly Better

Computers will be able to understand and produce American Sign Language (ASL) and other signed languages more accurately and comprehensively than they can today.[9] And eventually, they will exceed the abilities of most humans. With the advancements in computer vision and natural language processing, these systems are expected to become more accurate and robust. These advancements will lead to an environment where bidirectional recognition is not just a possibility but a norm. This means that not only will technology be adept at recognising ASL from users, but it will also effectively produce ASL or any other signed language, bridging the communication gap between those who communicate in a spoken language and those who use a sign language. It will also allow communication between people using different sign languages. This two-way interaction will play a pivotal role in making communication seamless for deaf and deaf–blind communities.

Static and Time-based Scene Analysis Will Be Comprehensive and Give Context-aware Responses – Allowing for Automated Generation of Visual and Audio Descriptions

Static scene analysis is the process of analysing a single image to identify objects, people and other features. **Time-based scene analysis** is the process of analysing a sequence of images to track the movement of objects and people over time.

Automated descriptions of static images are currently possible, although rudimentary today.[10,11,12] There are many applications in which automated descriptions, whether it is in Windows, iOS, Chrome or other offerings, have made a huge difference for people who are blind and have low vision.

Recently, significant advances in image processing algorithms have made it possible to extract more information from images. For example, MIT's Computer Science and Artificial Intelligence Laboratory (CSAIL) recently developed a Masked Generative Encoder (MAGE) – a system trainer to infer the missing parts of an image, which requires a deep understanding of the

image's content. Unlike other object identification and classification techniques, MAGE does not work with raw pixels. Instead, it converts images into
'semantic tokens' that abstract visual elements and come together to create
a simplified representation of an image. This representation can be used for
complex tasks while preserving the original image's information. This innovation has several applications such as improved object identification and
classification within images, faster learning from a small set of examples, the
creation of images under specific conditions like text or class and enhancement
of existing images (Li et al., 2023).

In the near future, computers will be able to analyse a scene and accurately
identify all of the objects in the scene as separate objects – with an understanding of their properties and functions.[13]

Inputs into Automated Systems (e.g., AI Systems, Chatbots) Will Go beyond Audio, Vision and Text to Include even Direct Brain Interfaces

There have been remarkable advances in **brain–computer interface** (BCI)
technology. Non-invasive BCIs use modalities such as electroencephalograms
(EEGs) to decipher neural signals, such as those responsible for neuromotor
control. BCI research has shown substantial promise for individuals who
have mobility disabilities or neurological disorders, such as cerebral palsy,
'locked-in' syndrome and paralysis[14]. For example, Synchron has developed
the first BCI – the Stentrode can be implanted without surgery and used for
people with paralysis to control devices such as computers, phones and wheelchairs.[15] Additionally, BCI technology has shown promise in text elicitation
for individuals with 'locked-in' syndrome – giving them the ability to 'write'
by merely thinking of letters, with the desired text materialising on the screen
(Rezvani et al., 2023).

In the upcoming years, it is expected that more non-invasive techniques for
brain interfaces will be introduced, accelerating both the special and general
use of direct brain interfaces.

Output Will Go beyond Audio, Vision and Text

In the future, just as with input, output will expand beyond audio, vision and
text. It will include vibrotactile sensations, haptics, and applications involving
temperature and pressure. While these advancements are currently in the
early stages and aimed at creating a more immersive experience in virtual and
augmented reality, there are additional uses as well. The introduction of con-

trolled pressure, for instance, has the potential to provide relief from anxiety or provide additional channels of information for individuals who are blind or deaf-blind.

Interfaces Will Be Much More Customisable at an Individual Level

We often present the world through interfaces that many cannot comprehend. For those who do not understand the interfaces on their daily devices, there is currently no solution. Companies present predefined interfaces for the most part, although some have interface options or adjustments. However, users are still stuck with the general interface paradigms set forth by the developers.

Pushing back on the idea that we must adapt to interfaces, instead, future **interfaces could adapt to us**. Imagine if, through simulated inputs or via programmatically driven API access and automation, users could tailor interfaces according to their unique needs. Consider the possibilities:

- A mediation layer exists, representing and acting on the user's behalf, ensuring that they can understand and use the interface they are presented with.
- If a user is unable to complete an action using the native interface, their digital assistant could step in and create one they could use.

An alternate (supplemental) approach to accessibility

What if Interfaces Adapted to Us Instead of the Other Way Around?

What if an **Info-Bot** with an **Individual User Interface Generator** (IUIG) could act as an intermediary between the user and any interface they encounter, ensuring that the user is presented with an interface they can understand and use? If they cannot understand/use the native interface on the device, the Info-Bot with an IUIG specific to that individual would step in to create an interface that would be useable and work in a familiar way for the individual – even if they were encountering a device for the first time (See Figure 5.1).

What is proposed is to create:

- a single, open-source intelligent agent – the **Info-Bot** – that can be pointed at any interface, and it would be able to understand and operate the interface as well as 50 per cent of the population. It would not be as smart as people – just as smart as the median person in figuring out that interface. The Info-Bot would then feed that information to an IUIG.

- a range of **IUIGs** that can take the information from the Info-Bot – and create an interface that is tailored to an individual – taking into consideration their abilities, limitations, knowledge, background, culture and preferences.

This approach would ensure that users consistently encounter familiar, consistent interfaces, regardless of the devices they encounter and have to interact with – making technology more accessible and intuitive for everyone.

Additionally, this approach can potentially reduce the industry's burden to understand and design for every type, degree and combination of disability, while increasing product accessibility from 3 per cent to near ubiquity.

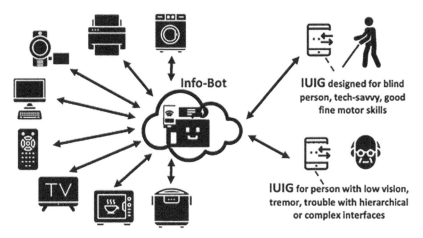

Figure 5.1   The Info-Bot and IUIG acting as an intermediary between user and interface

How It Would Work

Info-Bot

The Info-Bot would take any interface that it was exposed to, including an immersive 3D interface, and be able to understand and abstract it so that an alternate interface can be created that may be totally different (to meet user needs) but accomplishes the same functionality. For example, in the case of a user who is blind, a typical visual interface could be abstracted so that a completely optimised audio interface could be created from it by IUIGs.

(The output of the Info-Bot would be fed to the IUIG, which would create this alternate interface for the individual.)

Equipped with the capabilities of the median user, the Info-Bot could be exposed to any interface and perceive it just as an average human would – in other words, the Info-Bot would be able to see, hear and understand any controls, texts and visuals that the average (median) user is able to.

Some potential characteristics of the proposed Info-Bot are that it would:

- be free for all to use – as individuals – or for incorporation into product architectures;
- be able to understand interfaces at least as well as the 50th percentile human (the median):
  - Companies therefore would have to design a product that could be understood and used by at least half of the population (but no more) in order to have it understood by the Info-Bot;
  - If the Info-Bot could not understand some new feature of a company's product, the Info-Bot is open source, so the company can improve it so that it could;
- be open source (perhaps Lesser General Public License (LGPL)) so everyone can improve it and everyone can benefit from improvements. The LGPL is also important for compatibility and interoperability;
- be actively supported by industry and government(s) so it stays up to date and functioning at '50 per cent or better' level of the population;
- run in the cloud initially – but run locally in future;
- be separate from IUIGs initially but may merge with them later;
- be able to take output from the IUIGs and operate the product interface:
  - this may be via API or direct simulation of human control movements that the product is expecting;
- be maintained through government funding – or from industry as part of a social contract for industry being able to rely on the Info-Bot to address accessibility for those who cannot use the standard interface on their products.

IUIGs

IUIGs take the abstracted interface data from the Info-Bot and create an interface for an individual, at a particular time, and optimised for their abilities at that moment. This interface is not a transformation of the original interface into a different modality (i.e., it is not an auditory presentation of a visual interface like current screen readers). Rather, it is an interface that is completely optimised for that individual. It would be, for example, the interface that standard products would have if everyone in the world were exactly like this individual. If the individual is blind and not very good with technology, then the interface would be what products would have if everyone in the world were blind and not very good with technology. For an individual whose abilities change from day to day or even within the day, the ideal IUIG would change the interface presented to accommodate those changes.

Some characteristics of the envisioned IUIG would be that:

- each IUIG would be specific to an individual;
- for products with the same functionality but different interfaces, the IUIG would present the same (familiar, optimised) interface to the user – with just a different name:
    - for example, the user would see the same interface for all microwave ovens – with the only difference being features added or missing if they were present or missing from a particular microwave;
    - ditto for all TV streaming services. The choices, favourites, continue watching, search, sign in, etc., would all be presented and operate the same way;
    - if a TV streaming service changed its interface – the IUIG interface would not change unless there were new features – in which case they would be added to an interface that otherwise did not change;
- products with very different functionality would have different interfaces, but they would operate with user controls and metaphors that were familiar to the user;
- initially, IUIGs would be hand-designed by experts – individuals would select (or have selected for them) the IUIG that is best suited to their abilities and preferences;
- over time, AI could be used to help adapt and adjust IUIGs to be hyper-personalised for each individual user:
    - if an IUIG does not perfectly align with a user's needs, they would have the power to give feedback (e.g., 'That was too fast', or 'That was confusing', or 'Too many choices') and have their feedback used to refine and enhance the system. The focus here is on the individual's preferences and their lived experiences;
- all changes to the IUIG behaviour are under user control. This includes the ability to explore different IUIGs to see if they like other interface approaches better, and the ability to reject any change suggested:
    - similar to today's ATs, IUIGs would include both free versions and commercial versions;

– IUIGs that would account for different languages, cultures, etc., would also be available;

IUIGs would present the interface for any product the individual encounters in the form best suited to them. This may be visual, voice, tactile, simple, complex, few choices at a time, many choices at a time, using gestures, not requiring gestures, with large controls, with tiny controls requiring minimum movement, operable with eye-gaze, operable with thought, etc.

The key is that the individual would have an interface they could use with ANY product they encounter without the product manufacturer needing any understanding of their particular type, degree or combination of abilities/disabilities.

IUIGs could be created by AT vendors, researchers, consumers, family members, disability organisations, or anyone else with the skills required – to meet the needs of a person or people with different types, degrees and combinations of disabilities.

At first, IUIGs would likely resemble the current spectrum of interfaces provided by ATs. And they would leave the same gaps as our current ones do – reflecting our lack of understanding exactly how to design interfaces for many underserved groups. There are excellent general descriptions of the types of things that would help different underserved groups.[16] Later, as we carry out more research and develop targeted IUIGs for particular people in response to this new capability, a richer array of IUIGs will emerge that can address previously unaddressed and under-addressed users. The incorporation of AI may also allow us to address the problems presented by people whose abilities are changing rapidly – or whose abilities change from day to day or over the course of each day.

It is important to note that although the Info-Bot and the IUIGs would be separate in the beginning, they may eventually merge in order to provide a more optimum information exchange or tighter integration.

Benefits of the alternate approach

The benefits from such an approach would include benefits to users, product designers and government/society.

Benefits to Users

Some of the benefits to users would include near-total accessibility; universal compatibility; a unified interface for similar products; control over unsolicited changes; a standardised mental model; adaptability; addressing cognitive, language and learning needs; and reducing the learning curve.

Near-total accessibility: The IUIG and Info-Bot are major steps forward for accessibility. The accessibility gap would no longer be widening at an exponential rate, and accessibility would significantly increase from 3 per cent to 99 per cent – giving people with disabilities the same opportunities as everyone else for the first time. For those who struggle with technologies that they are forced to use in order to live independently – but cannot understand or use – this would be a sea change.

Universal compatibility The system is designed to work on all products everywhere and would offer consistent and instantaneous accessibility across devices and applications. It would not provide access to just one device but not another.

Unified interface for similar products: For products with the same or similar functions, users would need to learn only one interface. For example, let's say someone is trying to navigate a newly downloaded streaming services app (e.g., Netflix or Disney). All of these streaming services fundamentally offer the same functions (selecting and playing streamed content), but the user experience is drastically different for each. Every app presents its unique menu, navigation structure and interaction. Downloading a new one means the person has to learn a new interface despite the fact that it does basically (or identically) the same thing as the interface the user already knows. However, when using the Info-Bot/IUIG, instead of grappling with the different interfaces and confusing designs, the IUIG would offer the users a consistent and familiar experience that would work the same way for each service.

Control over unsolicited changes: Even if the interface of a product undergoes an update or change, the interface the IUIG would generate would remain unchanged for the user, offering a seamless experience. The system could prompt users to try out the new interface features – and even new interface approaches. But these would be offered and not forced, with the user able to accept, reject or accept and revert later to the old way, as they choose. Innovation would not be stifled, but rather unsolicited innovation would be managed. Preferably, any adaptation would be subtle and non-disruptive. One goal is to avoid solutions that users find irritating, like unsolicited and persistent help agents. Additionally, interfaces should not change abruptly. Even if the change is objectively 'better' (e.g., more efficient), some people prefer a certain way of doing things. In these cases, change can be the worst thing for them. The bottom line is user control of any unnecessary change.

Standardised mental model: Whether adjusting a thermostat, setting a microwave, or navigating a television interface, the user wouldn't have to juggle multiple interfaces and interactions. The IUIG would present familiar interface elements across the devices, whether it is pull-down menus or twisting dials, thus standardising an individual's user experience across different devices.

Adaptability: In the beginning, experts would design the initial user interfaces. However, as time progresses, while these interfaces might start off expert-designed, they could evolve to fit individual needs. For example, the interface might adjust accordingly as someone gains new skills. Conversely, if someone's abilities decline or if they are struggling due to ageing or other factors, the interface could adapt in different ways to accommodate those changes.

Addressing cognitive, language and learning needs: Our cognitive abilities are not static. They fluctuate, sometimes within moments. On some days, we may grasp concepts faster, while on others, we might need a little more time. We have all experienced moments of not understanding a concept until it is broken down for us or someone provides a concrete example. Then suddenly, we understand the concept more fully or in a more abstract or broad context. Especially with individuals who have cognitive, language and learning disabilities, presenting information at a lower understandable level first often enables them to then understand it in a higher-level presentation. With the Info-Bot, interfaces could start at a level the user understands and then gradually increase in complexity as a user grasps the concept – allowing every user to engage with technology effortlessly and equitably – simpler at first and more fully as they develop understanding.

Reducing the learning curve: Currently, many interfaces present a steep learning curve, leaving users feeling lost or overwhelmed. Users should not expend their mental energy navigating complicated interfaces. Instead, their focus should be solely on their intended task, be it content creation, communication, or any other endeavour. Just as with introducing content at a lower level and then raising it, IUIGs could start by using interface paradigms that are simpler or already familiar to the user when they encounter a new device or task. Then, as a person achieves skill and understands the task, more efficient interface elements could be introduced for adoption or rejection by the user.

Benefits to Industries

Some of the benefits to industry would include a decreased accessibility burden, a simplified design process, higher compliance and reduced litigation risks, scalability and wider market reach.

Decreased accessibility burden: The Info-Bot and IUIG would not require anyone – manufacturers, designers, developers, etc. – to have a deep understanding of accessibility or have disability expertise. This approach could also reduce the burden of constantly training staff due to organisational changes or turnover. Instead of depending on manufacturers, the mediation layer introduced by the Info-Bot/IUIG would be applied post-manufacture. In other words, after the product is already manufactured and in the user's hands, the Info-Bot/IUIG could provide access – by 'understanding' the product's interface and 'translating' it into a format the user can interact with based on their personal preferences and needs. This does not mean that companies should not continue to create products that are accessible out of the box for as many people as they can. It does mean, however, that they would be able to reach a much broader range of users – and have a safety net for those who have not been able to use their products, no matter how hard they have tried. This includes many who may not identify with having a disability – but simply find products too confusing or difficult to use.

Simplified design process: Designers could focus on what they do best without trying to learn and design for every type, degree and combination of disability. By providing a framework where the Info-Bot can intervene, they would still reach a broader audience.

Higher compliance and reduced litigation risks: Industries could achieve higher compliance levels in accessibility standards and prevent lawsuits. The current model is to build in as much accessibility for as many people in their team as is practical – and rely on ATs for those for whom built-in accessibility is not possible or practical. This same model can be extended to cover a much wider range of users by having the Info-Bot and IUIG act as a sort of super-AT to provide an alternate interface. However, instead of having the AT approach not available for closed products (where there is no API or programmatic access) the Info-Bot can achieve 'machine access' using only the standard human interface. Thus, with Info-Bot/IUIG, all products are accessible in the same way computers with screen readers are accessible to people who are blind.

Scalability and wider market reach: The Info-Bot and IUIG would be exponentially more scalable (to a wider range of users) than current accessibility approaches. The range of users who can use a product would be limited only by the availability of IUIGs for different types of users, and the ability of the use to understand the underlying function of the product (e.g., even if provided with an accessible interface, a person may not be able to understand a quantum computer sufficiently to operate it). Reaching a wider range of users – including those with multiple and cognitive disabilities common in older populations – can both increase profits but also improve the brand's reputation.

Benefits to Government/Society

The potential benefits to government and society include fewer regulations, fewer lawsuits and more people being able to participate in society.

Fewer regulations: Currently, accessibility guidelines and regulations go into great detail in order to try to make sure that all of the different aspects of products are accessible to as many types, degrees and combinations of disability as possible. As more and more kinds of ICT have emerged, including immersive technologies, and as more and more products are 'closed' (i.e., do not have a way for ATs to connect and work with them), the creation of accessibility standards has become more complicated and has put more and more requirements on industry to make these new technologies accessible. That is, where AT used to be able to be relied upon to provide access for many individuals with more severe disabilities, the lack of ability to use ATs with products means that companies need to provide those accessibility functions as a standard part of their product. This is very complicated to do. It is also very difficult to do for all types, degrees and combinations of disabilities. The result is both increasingly complex requirements, regulations and demands on industry and decreasing accessibility to users. An Info-Bot/IUIG approach would remove the need for many of these new requirements to provide built-in equivalents to ATs on closed products.

Fewer lawsuits – at least for ICTs: As accessibility becomes more complicated and difficult, the ability of companies to provide the same level of accessibility becomes more difficult and compliance may continue to be low or even reduce further. Creating a means for products with 'median' usability to be accessible could significantly reduce the effort needed by industry while greatly increasing the number of people who can use the products. The result would be fewer lawsuits (around ICT accessibility).

More people would be able to participate in society: There is both a fiscal and quality of life cost to society when people are not able to learn, work and live successfully and independently. As we build digital interfaces into more and more products and systems, we are putting them outside the understandability and operability of people who have trouble with or cannot use standard digital interfaces. To the extent that Info-Bot/IUIG can put these devices back within the reach of these people, we can increase the percentage of our population that is able to be successful in life and independent living.

What is needed to make this possible?

The concept is fairly simple, but what it requires is less so. Recent research and technological advancements hint at the feasibility of this vision. And we're already seeing projects that are laying the groundwork for it. In this section, we consider some of the advances that will be needed before this can be realised.

Abstracting User Interfaces

Abstracting user interfaces is an area of human–computer interaction (HCI) that focuses on designing interfaces in a way that separates the presentation of information from the underlying application functions. The idea is to allow for greater flexibility in presenting information to different users, on different devices, or in different contexts without having to redesign the entire application. Progress in this area includes ISO 24752 – a standard for a 'Universal Remote Console' (URC). The URC was an effort to standardise and abstract user interfaces so they can be easily personalised and adapted to different user needs and devices. ISO 24752 provides a framework for defining user interfaces in a way that separates the presentation and interaction from the underlying function of a device or service. However, one of the limitations of ISO 24752 is that it is impractical for every manufacturer and product designer to integrate a standard interface socket across their devices. Furthermore (and the primary reason that it failed), manufacturers were resistant to having someone 'control our product while looking at someone else's logo'. The Info-Bot/IUIG approach circumvents this and requires no API. However, the ISO 24752 work highlights the complexities of creating an abstract user interface socket – and something along this line will be required for communication between the Info-Bot and the IUIGs.

Artificial Intelligence

As modern interfaces increasingly merge visual, auditory and tactile elements, AI systems need to seamlessly integrate information from these multiple modalities. Advanced generative capabilities will be key for dynamic interface creation. But they do not 'understand' today so much as extrapolate from what has already been presented in the data they are built from. Significant advances in AI will be needed before it will be able to interpret and understand interfaces as well as the median human.

Understanding in Computer Vision

Beyond recognising objects or elements, machine vision systems must understand the context. For instance, distinguishing between a volume slider and a scroll bar is not just about their shapes but understanding their roles within the interface. Machine vision needs to move beyond pixel-level analysis and even object recognition to a more semantic understanding, extracting the meaning or intent behind visual elements.

Local Artificial Intelligence

AI technology is currently heavily cloud-based. However, with continual hardware advancements, it is increasingly heading towards being available locally rather than relying on servers in the cloud. Speech recognition, for example, has steadily moved from being cloud-based to locally based with an accompanying increase in user privacy. Using local AI would allow users to benefit from its capabilities without compromising their personal data.

Self-adaptation

As users interact with the Info-Bot, advancements in AI – specifically self-adaptation – will be needed to enable the intelligent agent to learn about the user's preferences and make changes accordingly – to change its behaviour or configuration in response to changes in the environment or new information.

User Interface Understanding

Understanding user interfaces (UIs) is core to developing the Info-Bot and IUIG. This involves applying computer vision and machine learning techniques to decipher the components of a UI without delving into its underlying structure. For example, if it's a graphical interface, you would have only pixels as input; for a voice interface, you would only have audio waveforms. The ability to derive the UI intent and functionality from just these inputs is an essential first step.

Apple has already taken steps in this direction with a product called Screen Recognition. This tool, an extension to the VoiceOver screen reader, helps navigate apps, through Infrastructure mode (i.e., if an app has included its metadata) or Screen Recognition mode (i.e., if the app does not have metadata). Users can activate the Screen Recognition mode to identify on-screen elements, facilitating easier navigation. However, one challenge lies in not just recognising these elements but understanding the user's intent. The next stage in UI understanding is discerning the tasks users want to accomplish.

Currently, machine learning models primarily that are trained to predict semantic UI information depend on datasets containing human-annotated static screenshots. However, this process is both expensive and error-prone for specific tasks. For instance, when annotators have to determine whether a UI element can be 'tapped' based on a screenshot, they must make educated guesses using visual cues alone. In response, Wu et al. have recently developed an automated mechanism to infer semantic properties of UIs. The Never-ending UI Learner is an app crawler that automatically examines apps obtained from a mobile app store and crawls them to infer semantic properties of UIs by interacting with UI elements, identifying and learning from different scenarios, and constantly updating the model based on this information (Wu et al., 2023).

Mapping User Intent into Actions

Unlike current assistants that require a specific command, such as Siri, advanced personal agents need to feature a dialogic interface. In other words, the assistant would use conversation or shared dialogue to understand meaning. It would be able to monitor in near-real-time and use natural language processing (NLP) to understand and act upon your intentions without you having to provide exact commands. For example, instead of saying, 'Raise the temperature', a user could express, 'I'm feeling cold', and the assistant would ask if they wanted to turn on the furnace or heat source. The ability to simply express one's feelings or state may suffice for the agent to decipher the necessary action to address some people's intent.

With today's technology, it is possible to map home automation technology to the appropriate assertions using AI. Consider an example from a YouTube video: a tech enthusiast spent an afternoon configuring ChatGPT as a shortcut on his iOS. This set-up allowed him to directly converse with ChatGPT, which then generated programmatic code to interact with his smart home. When he commented, 'I just noticed I'm sitting in the dark in my office', the system, without prompting or further interaction, turned on the lights. There was no need for a clarifying command or prolonged back-and-forth. Such an intuitive response demonstrates the growing capacity of AI-driven systems to map user statements to appropriate actions directly.[17] Given the trajectory of technological advancements, it is reasonable to anticipate that this level of automated comprehension and intent mapping will be even more sophisticated, widespread and commercially available two decades from now.

Content-based Understanding

Tasks such as 'summarise this chart for me' or 'turn these bullet points into a well-structured presentation' will be seamlessly handled by these systems. They will be capable of not just linguistic transformations but content-based transformations across various formats that are more accessible to some people.

In terms of knowledge queries, if one were to ask, 'Which restaurant did Gregg and I last dine at?', based on context, the system might enquire and ask to clarify, 'Which Gregg are you referring to?' If the response is 'Vanderheiden', the technology would recall that the last time you met with Gregg Vanderheiden was approximately five years ago in Seattle, pinpointing the exact restaurant from your calendar or charge card history.

These functionalities, though possible to some extent today in a pre-scripted manner, are predicted to be available automatically in the future, and this has implications as an assist and augmentative tool for several groups of people with disabilities or functional limitations, such as dementia or memory concerns, difficulties with visual processing or learning disabilities who may know what they want to accomplish with the product – but not understand how to operate its interface to achieve that result.

Multimodal Integration

Info-Bot and IUIGs would need to integrate and process diverse data streams, such as visual (from screens or interfaces), auditory (sounds, voice commands), tactile (touchscreen or hardware button feedback) and potentially more. Having a framework that can seamlessly bring together these varied data forms is invaluable. Currently, Microsoft Research is working on a project titled 'The Platform for Situated Intelligence', an open-source framework that alleviates the engineering challenges that arise when developing systems and applications that process multimodal streaming sensor data (such as audio, video, depth, etc.). The framework is intended to make it easier for developers to build AI that can perceive, understand and act in our world in real-time.[18]

Understanding How to Design an Interface for Each and Every Different Individual – with Their Different Types, Degrees and Combinations of Disability and Their Different Knowledge and Technical Abilities

Many of these research needs fall into the 'general ICT'/AI research realm. However, much research is also needed in understanding disability and adaptive interfaces. Developing the Info-Bot and IUIG will require a significant increase in our understanding of designing effective interfaces for people with *all* types, degrees and combinations of disabilities. This is especially important for people with multiple disabilities, as most ATs are designed for a single disability. For example, some ATs are designed for blind people, but they may not consider how blind people who also have another disability, such as deafness, cerebral palsy, or cognitive disabilities, would use their product. This can leave people with multiple disabilities without the AT they need. The more important problem, however, is that we do not actually know how to design products for people with all types, all degrees and all combinations of disabilities. Much research is needed to define the best or even adequate approaches for all of the permutations and combinations.

Automatic Generation of User Interfaces

Automatic generation of UIs is both an area of challenge and opportunity: opportunity since automatically generated interfaces are the core of the IUIGs. Any advances here will advance the development of IUIGs. However, IUIGs on mainstream products will pose a challenge to Info-Bots. Although Info-Bot's forte would be understanding any interface generated, it will be difficult for a company to determine that the Info-Bot can understand the interface(s) of their product – if the interfaces are generated after production and sale.

Back to the roots of the field?

It is interesting to note that most accessibility work began as efforts for individuals. In fact, most ATs on the market started out as something that was designed for an individual and then was generalised into a product.

Over time, the focus shifted to what is referred to today as 'universal design' or 'inclusive design'. That is building access directly into mainstream products for as many people as possible (with ATs filling in when it was not possible to build accessibility directly into products). This was followed by regulations requiring at least some minimum level of accessibility be built directly into products. For both AT and (even more so) mainstream products, the goal was to try to design for the widest range of people possible. In the context of AT, it was to cover the widest range of people with that particular disability. The result was products that were designed for people with 'typical' or 'average' or the 'most common' form of a disability.

More recently, a new approach has been championed that returns the field more to its roots. 'Ability-based design' focuses more on the individual and on creating general interfaces that can be adapted to a range of individual users (Wobbrock et al., 2018). Another approach characterised as 'solve for one – extend to many' is somewhat similar in that it focuses on the individual at the first stage and then tries to generalise that design to a broader range.

Hyper-personalisation and the use of IUIGs would seem to take us back to our roots – designing for one. Perhaps the ideal would indeed be the ability to create individual designs for each individual. Since it is not practical to do this manually, one person at a time, some mechanism for automating the process of creating individual UIs for each person, for each product they need to use, would seem to be the only way to achieve this.

Conclusions

Technology is often designed for a nominal user, who is typically young, is at least moderately digitally adept and has no disabilities. Despite increasing efforts to make technology more accessible, it is unlikely that we will ever reach a point where all technology is accessible to everyone out of the box. With new technologies rapidly being developed and current product accessibility as low as 3 per cent, it will be tremendously difficult to close the gap with traditional approaches that address the infrastructure layer. Today, a small subset of products is accessible to a subset of the range of disabilities and combinations of disabilities that people have.

Even if accessibility features are available, they are not always easy to use or understand, and some people with disabilities are excluded from using technology simply for this reason.

To make technology more accessible to everyone, we need to take a new approach that adapts the technology rather than demanding that individuals adapt to the technology. The Info-Bot and IUIG would dynamically generate accessible interfaces based on the user's needs, cognitive abilities, mobility, sensory perceptions and preferences. This approach has several advantages for users and industry, including achieving near-total accessibility, standardising a mental model, reducing industry burden and increasing scalability and profit.

The Info-Bot and IUIG have the potential to both address accessibility problems we are not able to address today for groups we do not serve well today and meet some of tomorrow's challenges as well. They also could provide a path for users, for the first time, to access all of the products created today without accessibility. They could provide accessibility if the company should have but did not implement accessibility. Even when required by law, accessibility is often not provided – but the Info-Bot/IUIG would still work. They also eliminate the problem that arises when the built-in accessibility is broken – but not repaired.

The feasibility, practicality and limitations of such an approach, however, are currently unknown – and a concerted R&D effort will be needed to explore this. This approach will also require developing a new social contract between product developers and consumers. It would also have a significant impact on policies and regulations around accessibility. Although the fundamental policies would not change, the implementing policies and regulations would need to change. Fortunately, it appears that it would simplify both the regulation and enforcement aspects. In addition, it would help address some of the emerging unsolved problems in accessibility regulation around both closed products and immersive environments, to name two. Further exploration of the concept is underway.[19]

Notes

1. Centers for Disease Control and Prevention, National Center on Birth Defects and Developmental Disabilities, Division of Human Development and Disability. Disability and Health Data System (DHDS) Data [online] [accessed 27 August 2023]. https://dhds.cdc.gov.
2. https://jimthatcher.com/index-old.htm.
3. https://www.apple.com/accessibility/.
4. https://trace.umd.edu/design-of-html-mosaic-pages-to-increase-their-accessibility-to-users-with-disabilities-strategies-for-today-and-tomorrow/.

5.   https://www.w3.org/WAI/GL/central.htm.
6   https://www.reuters.com/technology/chatgpt-sets-record-fastest-growing-user
     -base-analyst-note-2023-02-01/.
7   https://www.bemyeyes.com.
8   rewordify.com.
9   'First' SL real-time general/public use translator. https://www.slait.ai/.
10   https://support.google.com/chrome/answer/9311597?hl=en&co=GENIE
     .Platform%3DDesktop.
11   https://blogs.windows.com/msedgedev/2022/03/17/appears-to-say-microsoft
     -edge-auto-generated-image-labels/.
12   https://www.apple.com/accessibility/vision/.
13   https://futureofinterface.org/auditorium_cpt/machine-computer-vision/.
14   https://time.com/6298543/paralysis-reversal-keith-thomas/.
15   https://synchron.com/.
16   Making Content Usable for People with Cognitive and Learning Disabilities W3C
     Working Group Note 29 April 2021. https://www.w3.org/TR/coga-usable/.
17   https://www.youtube.com/watch?v=THeet9bbphw.
18   https://www.microsoft.com/en-us/research/project/platform-situated
     -intelligence/.
19   For more information, see https://info-bot.org/.

References

Borsos, Z., Marinier, R., Vincent, D., Kharitonov, E., Pietquin, O., Sharifi, M., Roblek, D., Teboul, O., Grangier, D., Taliasacchi, M., & Zeghidour, N. (2023). AudioLM: A language modeling approach to audio generation. *IEEE/ACM Transactions on Audio, Speech, and Language Processing, 31,* 2523–2533. DOI:10.1109/TASLP.2023.3288409

Copeland, K. (1974). *Aids for the Severely Handicapped.* Grune & Stratton.

Keates, S. (2006). SIGACCESS member profile: Jim Thatcher. *ACM SIGACCESS Accessibility and Computing, 85,* 56–56.

Lazar, J., Jordan, J.B., & Vanderheiden, G. (2019). Toward unified guidelines for kiosk accessibility. *Interactions, 26*(4), 74–77.

Li, T., Chang, H., Mishra, S., Zhang, H., Katabi, D., & Krishnan, D. (2023). Mage: Masked generative encoder to unify representation learning and image synthesis. *Proceedings of the IEEE/CVF Conference on Computer Vision and Pattern Recognition* (pp. 2142–2152). DOI:10.1109/CVPR52729.2023.00213

Rezvani, S., Hosseini-Zahraei, S., Tootchi, A., Guger, C., Chaibakhsh, Y., Saberi, A., & Chaibakhsh, A. (2023). A review on the performance of brain-computer interface systems used for patients with locked-in and completely locked-in syndrome. *Cognitive Neurodynamics.* https://doi.org/10.1007/s11571-023-09995-3

Schauer, J., Novak, M., & Vanderheiden, G.C. (1994). General input device emulating interface (GIDEI) standard. *Journal of Rehabilitation Research and Development, 30–31,* 150. https://www.proquest.com/scholarly-journals/general-input-device-emulating-interface-gidei/docview/215284876/se-2

Schwejda, P., & Vanderheiden, G. (1982). Adaptive-firmware card for the Apple II [input for physically disabled]. *Byte, 7*(9), 276–314. http://archive.org/stream/byte-magazine

-1982 -09 -rescan/ 1982_09_BYTE_07-09_Computers_and_the_Disabled#page/ n277/mode/2up

Spitale, G., Biller-Andorno, N., & Germani, F. (2023). AI model GPT-3 (dis)informs us better than humans. *Science Advances, 9*, DOI:10.1126/sciadv.adh1850

Vanderheiden, G., Lazar, J., Lazar, A., Kacorri, H., & Jordan, J.B. (2022). *Technology and Disability: 50 Years of Trace R&D Center Contributions and Lessons Learned.* Springer Nature.

Vanderheiden, G.C. (1983). *Curbcuts and Computers: Providing Access to Computers and Information Systems for Disabled Individuals.* Trace Center. https://files.eric.ed .gov/fulltext/ED289314.pdf

Vanderheiden, G.C. (1981). Practical application of microcomputers to aid the handicapped. *Computer, 14*(1), 54–61. DOI:10.1109/C-M.1981.220173

Vanderheiden, G.C., & Grilley, K. (Eds.) (1976). *Non-vocal Communication Techniques and Aids for the Severely Physically Handicapped.* University Park Press.

Vanderheiden, G.C., Volk, A.M., & Geisler, C.D. (1973). The auto-monitoring communication board (AutoCom). A new communication aid for the severely handicapped. *Proceedings of the 1973 Carnahan Conference on Electronic Prosthetics* (pp. 47–51). University of Kentucky, Office of Research and Engineering Services.

Wobbrock, J.O., Gajos, K.Z., Kane, S.K., & Vanderheiden, G.C. (2018). Ability-based design. *Communications of the ACM, 61*(6), 62–71. https://doi.org/10.1145/3148051

Wu, J., Krosnick, R., Schoop, E., Swearngin, A., Bigham, J.P., & Nichols, J. (2023). Never-ending learning of user interfaces. *arXiv preprint*. https://arxiv.org/pdf/2308 .08726.pdf

6. A UK example of the relationship between ATech research and ATech policy

Robert McLaren, Shamima Akhtar and Clive Gilbert

Introduction

The authors of this chapter are all policy professionals at Policy Connect which is a UK-based cross-party think tank. We provide the secretariat for the All-Party Parliamentary Group for Assistive Technology, which raises the profile of assistive technology (ATech) within Parliament and delivers the ATech Policy Lab, a partnership with Bournemouth University and the Ace Centre charity whose mission is to design public policy so that technology works for everyone. We draw on academic research and expertise to inform our work including briefings to policy makers, consultation responses, and reports that make recommendations to policy makers.

As policy professionals we have a particular interest in the contribution of academic research on technology and disability to the UK government's policy making processes. Similarly, and looking at things from the other direction, we are interested in how public policy can support academic work on ATech. Indeed, one would hope that the efforts of policy makers and researchers together form a virtuous cycle: government funds research on ATech, which then informs better policy making on ATech, including better targeting of research funding towards the most important issues related to ATech and disability. For example, a study of disabled people's experiences with care robots might inform new clinical guidance and help demonstrate the need for an innovation project to address the issues that end-users identified with existing robots. Of course, not all ATech research needs to inform policy, and research funding policy should not be over-prescriptive about the direction of ATech research. But it is desirable that research and public policy around technology and disability form a mutually improving relationship.

In this chapter we seek to provide a picture of the current relationship between research and policy in the ATech field by investigating what kinds of evidence the UK government cites in its policy statements on ATech. We then make some observations regarding the picture that emerges from this exercise. Finally, we make some recommendations to promote the better utilisation of government-funded academic ATech research by policy makers.

The UK National Disability Strategy as an example of UK policy makers' use of ATech research

The National Disability Strategy (HM Government, 2021) is one of just two commitments on disability in the 2019 Conservative manifesto (the other being on accessible housing), and it aimed to be 'the most far-reaching endeavour in this area for a generation or more'. Disability groups were generally critical of the strategy for failing to meet its stated ambition and of the way the strategy was developed without, it was claimed, adequate involvement of disabled people.[1] Nonetheless, it remains significant for its cross-departmental approach and, with respect to ATech, for its several commitments on the topic and for its announcement of a new ambition 'to help make the UK the most accessible place in the world to live and work with technology'. For example, the Strategy committed to 'invest up to £1 million in 2021 to 2022 to develop a new Centre for Assistive and Accessible Technology, reporting on progress by summer 2022', which was welcomed by disability groups.

The Strategy also committed to a number of actions on technology that have already been delivered. For example, the Strategy said government would 'assess the assistive and accessible technology needs of disabled people in England', and this work was commissioned and has now been published (see Austin et al., 2023). The Strategy also said government would 'explore how to improve the accessibility of private sector websites', and we understand that the government's Open Innovation Team have produced an internal government report on this topic. The Strategy also aimed to 'tackle the Accessibility Skills Gap', and subsequent work on this topic has brought about the publication of guidance on the role of accessibility specialists within government (see Central Digital and Data Office, 2022).

We therefore suggest that by investigating policy makers' use of ATech research in the Strategy we can get a picture – if only a snapshot – of the relationship between policy and research in this area.

Findings

In examining how the National Disability Strategy used UK-funded ATech research to justify or underpin its proposed commitments we will first look at direct (primary) citations of academic research. We will then explore secondary citations of academic research (citations within citations). To be counted as UK ATech research that has informed the Strategy, we required that the cited research mention technology, but we did not discount works that were positioned in a section within the document that was unrelated to technology.[2]

Primary Citations of Academic Research in the UK National Disability Strategy

The Strategy cites 14 outputs in its discussion of ATech. Of these, six were reports from NGOs (Non-Governmental Organisations), three were the government's own outputs and five were academic studies (Edyburn, 2020; Luckin et al., 2020; Quintero, 2022 Seale, 2020; WebAIM, 2020). Of these academic studies, three appear to have been supported in some way by UK government funding: Seale (2020), Edyburn (2020) and Luckin et al. (2020). Professor Jane Seale is affiliated with a UK Higher Education Institution (the Open University) that receives state funding; Edyburn (2020) was commissioned by the Department of Education; and Luckin et al. (2020) were commissioned by the Council for Science and Technology. In what follows, we refer to academic studies whose production has been in some way supported by UK government funding as 'UK academic research' as a shorthand.

How should we assess whether the use of these three papers represents an adequate degree of engagement between policy making and UK research? The government publishes an annual *Assistive technology research and development report*, describing the research that the government has funded to improve equipment that enables independence or well-being of disabled and older people (this is a requirement made by Section 22 of the Chronically Sick and Disabled Persons Act 1970[3]). During the period when the National Disability Strategy was being developed (January 2020–July 2021) the most recent research and development report listed 150 active projects,[4] and the Strategy itself reports that in 2019 to 2020, UK Research and Innovation (UKRI) invested £58.4 million "in research and development related to assistive technology" (HM Government, 2021, p. 76).

Given this level of UK ATech research activity, the Strategy's three citations of such work (out of 14 total citations on ATech) does appear rather low. It appears, in other words, that there is a disconnect between policy making and research: either policy makers are underutilising the work they fund, or much of current research is not relevant to policy making (or both). However, perhaps this appearance is misleading. It might be that the policy makers behind the National Disability Strategy have made use of UK research by reviewing and citing works that themselves synthesise a wide range of UK research outputs. For example, the Strategy asserts the 'importance of involving disabled consumers in the design process' and cites just one review paper, Quintero (2022). This is perhaps a sensible approach, making use of a single (recent) review of the evidence around participatory design, rather than citing dozens of studies that each addresses some niche within the field. Although Quintero is affiliated to two Colombian universities, the review makes use of UK academic research to form its broad conclusions about the value of participatory design. If this is true more broadly – i.e., if the Strategy cites works that themselves make significant use of UK academic research – then we can say that UK academic research has indeed informed the strategy.[5]

Secondary Citations of Academic Research in the UK National Disability Strategy

In this section we will examine what UK academic research is cited by those publications that are directly cited in the Strategy.

Citations within NGO reports

The majority of the six NGO reports cited by the Strategy contain primary research, consisting of surveys and other data recording disabled people's views. The papers that also cite other research mostly cite other NGOs and government outputs. There are a total of 17 citations of academic outputs in the NGO reports, of which 10 could be counted as UK research (given that one or more author is affiliated with a UK Higher Education Institution). Of the ten UK research outputs cited by NGO reports, eight explicitly mentioned technology and so can be counted as UK ATech research. An example of a secondary citation that did not explicitly mention technology is the report by the charity Leonard Cheshire entitled *Reimagining the Workplace* (Leonard Cheshire, 2019). The National Disability Strategy cites *Reimagining the Workplace* because the report argues that ATech is vital for disability inclusion in the workplace. However, the report only cites one example of UK research, and this citation appears in a section where ATech is not mentioned. Furthermore, the paper in question (Dwyer, 2018) does not mention 'technology' (or its common analogies).

Citations within government outputs

Three government outputs were cited in the Strategy. One was published by the Centre for Data Ethics and Innovation. This cites five outputs in connection with disability, but none are academic in nature: one is an NGO report, the others are newspaper and magazine articles. The second report is the government's guidance on the public sector web accessibility requirements, which cites no academic work (although it does cite an NGO report and private sector report). The third report is the government's response to a consultation on electric vehicle charging, which similarly does not cite any academic work.

Citations within academic outputs

The five academic outputs cited in the Strategy cited 20 UK ATech outputs. WebAIM (2020) cited no other works; Quintero (2022) cited four UK ATech academic outputs; Seale (2020) cited four UK ATech academic outputs; Luckin et al. (2020) cited six UK ATech academic outputs; and Edyburn (2020) cited six UK ATech academic outputs.

In summary, the National Disability Strategy cited five academic ATech research publications, of which three were funded by the UK government. The Strategy cited 14 works in total, which in turn cited a further 28 UK academic ATech outputs.

Discussion

In this section we will make some observations about the commonalities of the particular works cited by the Strategy and consider the limitations of the methodology.

Observations

Now that we have identified the particular works that have informed the Strategy, we offer three observations about their commonalities:

1. *Open*: with the exception of Quintero (2022), all the ATech academic outputs cited by the Strategy are available online without a paywall or log-in. In addition, when we turn to the NGO reports and government reports cited by the Strategy, we find that these in turn are often cited ATech academic outputs that are freely available. This may reflect policy

makers' lack of access to academic journals and/or the use of standard search engines to discover work (see Goodes and Broadley, 2022).

2. *Recent*: it is striking that the Strategy's oldest citation on ATech is a report from 2018 and all the academic citations were from 2020, the year during which the Strategy began to be developed. This may reflect a view among policy makers that technology development is so rapid as to make findings quickly obsolete – a view that may or may not be correct.

3. *Broad in scope*: of the five academic studies that were directly cited, three were literature reviews. As we suggested earlier, policy makers may regard these kinds of studies as an efficient way to evidence the broad claims that need to be made to justify policy initiatives – e.g., evidencing the claim that ATech can be helpful for autistic people.

Limitations of Methodology

One limitation of this exercise is that it involves making choices of definition which are not self-evident or uncontroversial. For example, someone might define an academic output as one that has a Digital Object Identifier, and this would rule out several works we have counted. We have tried to be explicit about the definitional choices we have made so that readers can judge their reasonableness. A related problem is that we lack all the information we would need to definitively determine whether a given work was supported by UK research funding, and so have used author affiliation as a proxy: we can see that this opens up the possibility of inaccurate counting (for example, Dave Edyburn is not affiliated with a UK institution but his work was funded by the UK government directly).

A second limitation is that we only considered the National Disability Strategy and this of course may be an outlier. However, a less formal survey of other significant documents such as *People at the Heart of Care* (2021), the *Special Educational Needs and Disabilities (SEND) and Alternative Provision (AP) Improvement Plan* (2023), the House of Lords' briefing 'Assistive technology in education and employment' (2023), and the Parliamentary Office of Science and Technology paper 'Invisible Disabilities in Education and Employment' (2023) suggest a similar pattern of citations.[6,7,8,9]

Recommendations for increasing the use of ATech research by policy makers

Based on our examination of how the National Disability Strategy utilised UK ATech research we have two main recommendations: (1) make research more discoverable and (2) fund and support broader-based research.

Make Research More Discoverable

As we noted earlier, policy makers appear to value research that is easy to find and is up to date. We suggest that government use its existing practice of publishing annual 'Assistive technology research and development [R&D] reports' to help satisfy this preference (see DHSC, 2023). These reports are published annually to comply with Section 22 the Chronically Sick and Disabled Persons Act 1970. Each annual report 'sets out government-funded projects supporting the development, introduction and evaluation of assistive technology'. If these reports included a searchable (e.g., coded with tags) collection of the years' ATech research outputs, they would provide an obvious starting place for policy makers looking for evidence on ATech. The R&D reports are themselves freely available and highly discoverable (being on the government website and, more recently, published in HTML) so even if the outputs listed in the reports are not freely available, the reports would still help make the existence of those works visible.

However, the R&D reports do not currently serve as an effective starting point for policy makers looking for evidence on ATech. For the most part, the reports do not link to published outputs. Instead the reports catalogue active or recently completed projects; that is, the reports function (as intended) as a review investment in UK ATech research but not as a guide to the outputs from that investment. In addition, the R&D reports are incomplete even as surveys of government-funded research projects. Firstly, because their methodology is to canvas research funding councils for the work they are supporting, the reports undercount the work funded by other government bodies and undercount projects that are not the result of a targeted funding council award. Of the examples of UK ATech research cited in the National Disability Strategy, only Edyburn (2020) is referenced in R&D reports. In contrast, Luckin et al. (2020), which was funded by the Government Office for Science, is missing from the relevant reports – as are other similar outputs such as the NHSX Adult Social Care Technology and Digital Skills Review[10] and the Government Digital Service's report from its monitoring of website accessibility.[11] The absence of Seale (2020) from the R&D reports shows that even work which makes a substantial impact (being used by policy makers to help design and support the case for a £2.5 million Digital Lifeline Fund) may not be included as it was not tied to a specific funding council award. Secondly, while the defined scope of the R&D reports is broad (counting research on 'any product or service designed to enable independence for disabled and older people') the reports appear, in practice, to be dominated by research on medical-adjacent products and interventions as opposed to, for example, ATech that is used in the workplace (this is our impression which is hard to show by objective measures, but it is notable that in the most recent report the word 'treatment' appears 14 times while words associated with employment are only used once when referring to disabled people – and three times when referring to the careers of researchers and clinicians). This, no doubt, reflects the funding decisions of research councils which may favour medical-adjacent work, but it is also likely that the R&D reports are missing some of the non-medical research that is funded by government. For example, dyslexia is a high-incidence specific learning difficulty around which we expect there is some active research connected to technology, and yet the words 'dyslexic' or 'dyslexia' do not appear in the most recent R&D report at all.

The aforementioned observations suggest a reform to the R&D reports process that would make them both more complete and accurate surveys of research funding (their current purpose) and make the reports a resource for policy makers, leading to greater use of UK ATech academic research in policy. We propose that a process should be created so that researchers can submit their ongoing projects and published works to the R&D reports team for possible inclusion in the report (the submission form could also invite researchers to choose tags for their project or output, such as 'muscular skeletal', 'AI', 'education', 'digital', 'literature review', etc.). Academics would have an incentive to do this as it would make their work more discoverable, including by policy makers. In addition, civil service researchers (such as Government Digital Service) would adopt such reporting as part of their standard project delivery. The submissions system would have to be supported by additional resources to the R&D reports team, but we would argue that this small spend is easily justified to ensure that ATech research achieves greater impact, and so enable government's nine-figure annual spending on such research to achieve greater value for money. It may also be wise to move the responsibility for delivering the R&D reports from the Department for Health and Social Care to the Government Office for Science to mitigate biases toward research on medical-adjacent research.

These observations about discoverability also suggest that, even without the reforms we propose here, researchers should consider how to enable their work to be more easily seen by policy makers. In our experience, a good approach is to publish non-technical blogs that reference one's published research, as these will show up in search results (including queries by AI search bots). For example, when we were exploring the scope of the then incoming web accessibility requirements for public sector bodies, we found a blog from Dr Albert Sanchez-Graells that wrote up the findings from his and Andrea Gideon's paper on whether universities count as public sector bodies. We then engaged with both Dr Gideon and Dr Sanchez-Graells and used their paper and wider expertise to inform policy making on the topic of the scope of the incoming web accessibility regulations.[12,13]

Fund and Support Broader-based Research

We noted in the observations section that policy makers appear to value research that makes broad conclusions, as opposed to being concerned with a particular product in a particular setting. The reforms to the R&D reports we suggested earlier would give us a clearer picture of which kinds of ATech research (topics, disciplines, approaches) are currently favoured. Reviewing this may show a comparative lack of this broad-based research, or we may find that ATech research of this broader sweep abounds but is obscure to policy makers for the reasons we also explored in the 'Observations' section. Nonetheless, given the value that policy makers place on broader-based research – literature reviews, meta-analyses, and single studies on wide topics such as website accessibility (see WebAIM, 2020) – we propose that research funders and researchers themselves consider how work of this kind can be better supported and rewarded.

It is also possible that there is simply too little funding for ATech research as a whole, leaving policy makers too little work to draw upon. We note that the Work and Pensions Select Committee, in 2018, recommended the introduction of an ATech 'grand challenge' in the Industrial Strategy but this proposal was rejected by the government on the grounds that the existing Ageing Society Grand Challenge would fund work on ATech but it is unclear how much research on ATech has been funded by that Challenge.[14]

Conclusions

In this chapter we used the National Disability Strategy as a case study to illuminate how the UK government draws on UK ATech research in its policy statements. Our analysis suggests that the use of UK-funded ATech research by policy makers is currently rather limited. We therefore recommend that UK ATech research needs to be made more discoverable and potentially include more broad-based studies. To contribute towards fulfilling the recommendations we have made, the ATech Policy Lab will publish an annual review of the UK research on ATech outputs that were funded by government departments and public bodies other than research councils. We hope that this will demonstrate the value of the more comprehensive reforms to the R&D research reports process that we recommend (and we will happily give over this task to the Office for Science should our recommendations be taken up).

Notes

1   In July 2023 the UK government won its appeal. It made a statement on what this means for delivery of the National Disability strategy in September 2023. See: https://commonslibrary.parliament.uk/research-briefings/cbp-9599/.

2   We made one exception for the Centre for Data Ethics and Innovation paper 'Bias in Algorithmic Decision Making', which is available from: https://www.gov.uk/government/publications/cdei-publishes-review-into-bias-in-algorithmic-decision-making. This is not a study about disability or accessibility, and it cites approximately 261 works. Our approach in this case was to review all the citations the study made in the short passage at which it considered disability.

3   Section 2 of the Chronically Sick and Disabled Persons Act 1970: https://www.legislation.gov.uk/ukpga/1970/44/section/22.

4   Research and development work relating to assistive technology 2018 to 2019. https://www.gov.uk/government/publications/research-and-development-work-relating-to-assistive-technology-2018-to-2019.

5   For example, Quintero (2022) cites Nasr et al. (2016). Several of the authors of this publication are affiliated to UK institutions, including the University of Sheffield and the University of Hertfordshire.

6   *People at the Heart of Care: Adult Social Care Reform White Paper* (2021): https://www.gov.uk/government/publications/people-at-the-heart-of-care-adult-social-care-reform-white-paper.

7   *The Special Educational Needs and Disabilities (SEND) and Alternative Provision (AP) Improvement Plan* (2023): https://www.gov.uk/government/publications/send-and-alternative-provision-improvement-plan.

8   The House of Lords' briefing 'Assistive technology in education and employment' (2023): https://lordslibrary.parliament.uk/assistive-technology-in-education-and-employment/.

9   Parliamentary Office of Science and Technology paper 'Invisible Disabilities in Education and Employment' (2023): https://post.parliament.uk/research-briefings/post-pn-0689/.

10   NHSX Adult Social Care Technology and Digital Skills Review (2021): https://www.ipsos.com/en-uk/nhsx-reviews-published-digital-technology-innovation-and-digital-skills-adult-social-care.

11   Government guidance on public sector websites and mobile application accessibil-
     ity monitoring: https://www.gov.uk/guidance/public-sector-website-and-mobile
     -application-accessibility-monitoring.
12   See the blogs by Sanchez-Graells (2016), 'Can English universities adopt a more
     commercial approach and stop complying with EU public procurement law?'
     (https://legalresearch.blogs.bris.ac.uk/2016/04/can-english-universities-adopt-a
     -more-commercial-approach-and-stop-complying-with-eu-public-procurement
     -law/) and Sanchez-Graells (2018), 'UK Universities must soon comply with the
     EU Web Accessibility Directive' (https://legalresearch.blogs.bris.ac.uk/2018/07/uk
     -universities-must-soon-comply-with-the-eu-web-accessibility-directive/).
13   See the paper by Gideon and Albert Sanchez-Graells (2015) 'When are universi-
     ties bound by EU public procurement rules as buyers and providers? – English
     universities as a case study': https://papers.ssrn.com/sol3/papers.cfm?abstract_id
     =2692966.
14   One programme funded by the Industrial Strategy Challenge Fund (ISCF) to
     support the Ageing Society Grand Challenge is the Healthy Ageing Challenge,
     which has spent £98 millon to date. The 2022 'UKRI Healthy Ageing Challenge:
     Our Story So Far' report does mentiontwo projects that involved ATech ('Healthy
     Homes, Healthy Lives' and 'Disabled Living').

References

Austin, V., Patel, D., Danemayer, J., Mattick, K., Landre, A., Smitova, M., Banduka, M.,
    Healy, A., Chockalingam, N., Bell, D., & Holloway, C. (2023). *Assistive Technology
    Changes Lives: An Assessment of AT Need and Capacity in England.* Cabinet Office,
    HMG. https:// www . disability innovation .com/ publications/ at -country -capacity
    -england
Central Digital and Data Office (2022). *Guidance: Accessibility Specialist.* https://www
    .gov.uk/guidance/accessibility-specialist
DHSC (Department of Health and Social Care) (2023). Collection: Assistive Technology
    Research and Development Reports. https://www.gov.uk/government/collections/assistive
    -technology-research-and-development-reports#full-publication-update-history
Dwyer, P. (2018). *Final Findings Report: The Welfare Conditionality Project 2013–2018.*
    University of York. https:// eprints .whiterose .ac .uk/ 154305/ 1/ 1 ._FINAL_Welfare
    _Conditionality_Report_complete.pdf
Edyburn, D. (2020). *Rapid Literature Review on Assistive Technology in Education.*
    https://assets.publishing.service.gov.uk/government/uploads/system/uploads/
    attachment_data/file/937381/UKAT_FinalReport_082520.pdf
Goodes, H., & Broadley, S. (2022). Increasing the Impact of Research through
    Policy: The Role of Academic Publishers in Bringing Researchers and Policymakers
    Together. In R. Iphofen & D.O. Mathúna (Eds.), *Ethical Evidence and Policymaking:
    Interdisciplinary and International Research* (pp. 347–364). Bristol University Press.
    https://doi.org/10.51952/9781447363972.ch018
HM Government (2021). *The National Disability Strategy.* https:// www .gov .uk/
    government/publications/national-disability-strategy

Leonard Cheshire (2019). *Reimagining the Workplace: Disability and Inclusive Employment.* https://www.leonardcheshire.org/sites/default/files/2020–02/reimagining-the-workplace-disability-inclusive-employment.pdf

Luckin, R., Blake, C., Kent, C., & Clarke-Wilson, A. (2020). Technology-led Interventions for SpLDs. In *Current Understanding, Support Systems, and Technology-led Interventions for Specific Learning Difficulties: Evidence Reviews Commissioned for Work by the Council for Science and Technology.* https:// assets .publishing .service .gov .uk/ government/ uploads/ system/ uploads/ attachment _data/ file/ 926052/ specific -learning-difficulties-spld-cst-report.pdf

Quintero, C. (2022). A review: Accessible technology through participatory design. *Disability & Rehabilitation: Assistive Technology, 17*(4), 369–375. [Published online 3 July 2020]. DOI:10.1080/17483107.2020.1785564

Seale, J. (2020). Keeping connected and staying well: The role of technology in supporting people with learning disabilities during the coronavirus pandemic. The Open University. https://oro.open.ac.uk/75127/

WebAIM (2020). *The WebAIM Million: An Analysis of the Top 1,000,000 Home Pages* https://webaim.org/projects/million/

7. Rethinking assistive technology research and the evidencing of assistive technology outcomes

Dave Edyburn

Introduction

The field of assistive technology (AT) has evolved considerably over the past 40 years. Three pillars are notable for understanding the drivers of change during this period: policy, innovative product development and research (Scherer et al., 2019; Edyburn, 2013). In this chapter, I will describe the evolution of AT in the context of the United States and will offer observations about how the developments are similar/different in the context of the global adoption of AT. More importantly, I will argue that while all three pillars will continue to be essential for propelling the field forward, it will be the research pillar that has the most potential for transformative change, particularly in relation to evidencing the outcomes of AT use.

Futurist Alan Kay offered a provocative change strategy when he said, 'The best way to predict the future is to invent it.' To that end, I will offer a series of suggestions for rethinking AT research in order to establish a robust system of AT outcome evidence. Such a vision will require considerable technical innovation in order to automate AT data collection and analysis. In particular, the AT profession will need to collaborate with data scientists in order to utilise machine learning (ML), data analytics and artificial intelligence (AI) techniques that will optimise performance through the AT-human interface. The scenarios presented may be helpful for defining individual and shared research agendas in anticipation of a future that may be vastly different than the recent past.

Background: Understanding the Field of Assistive Technology

Before providing an overview of what I regard to be the pillars that are driving change in the AT field, some background context will be provided.

The need for AT

At the present time, there is no agreed upon definition, or universal assessment instrument, for determining who needs AT or how one might benefit. As a result, AT advocates must be aware of observational characteristics indicating that an AT evaluation might be worthwhile when a person fails to complete a key life task and/or routine tasks are distinguished by many negative attributes such as excessive time to complete, significant frustration and/or poor quality of the end-product. There is an unknown population of individuals who could benefit from AT if they were merely introduced to the possibilities and subsequently provided appropriate AT devices and services.

AT devices and services

In the US, in the context of educational provision for children, 'Assistive technology device' means any item, piece of equipment, or product system, whether acquired commercially off the shelf, modified or customised, that is used to increase, maintain or improve the functional capabilities of a child with a disability (U.S. Department of Education, 2006, 2011). Some experts have argued that the definition of AT is so broad that it could include anything (Edyburn, 2003). In fact, that is a simple way to think about it: AT is anything that improves the functional performance of an individual with a disability. This perspective of AT devices is encompassing in terms of possibilities but frustrating for administrators and funders who must adjudicate requests for AT provision.

In US federal law, 'Assistive technology service' means any service that directly assists a child with a disability in the selection, acquisition or use of an assistive technology device.[1] Such a term includes:

a. The evaluation of the needs of a child with a disability, including a functional evaluation of the child in the child's customary environment.
b. Purchasing, leasing or otherwise providing for the acquisition of assistive technology devices by children with disabilities.
c. Selecting, designing, fitting, customising, adapting, applying, maintaining, repairing or replacing assistive technology devices.

d. Coordinating and using other therapies, interventions or services with assistive technology devices, such as those associated with existing education and rehabilitation plans and programmes.

e. Training or technical assistance for a child with a disability or, where appropriate, the family of such child; and

f. Training or technical assistance for professionals (including individuals providing education or rehabilitation services), employers or other individuals who provide services to, employ or are otherwise substantially involved in the major life functions of such child.

AT outcomes and outcome measurement systems

In focus group research conducted by the Assistive Technology Outcomes Measurement System (ATOMS) Project, AT service directors identified a list of variables that might be measured to understand the outcomes associated with AT use: (1) change in performance/function (body, structure, activity), (2) change in participation, (3) usage and why or why not, (4) consumer satisfaction (process, devices), (5) goal achievement, (6) quality of life, (7) cost, (8) demographics, (9) AT interventions (services and devices) and (10) environmental context.[2] This list raises significant questions about whether or not AT outcomes are a single or multifaceted variable as well as who determines which outcome is most important (Rust & Smith, 2006; Edyburn, 2002).

Measuring the outcomes of assistive technology must address the user, the AT device and the AT service delivery system. Furthermore, the "evaluation process in the service delivery system [must be] designed to measure and establish a baseline of what works; how well something works; for which clients it works; and at what level of economic efficiency it works" (DeRuyter, 1997, p. 90).

AT stakeholders

Stakeholders are all the people who have a vested interest in a policy. In the context of AT, the key stakeholders are the individual with a disability, parents/family, teachers/employers, assistive technology specialists, occupational therapists, speech language therapists, developers, vendors and payers (i.e., insurance companies, government). Research has demonstrated that change initiatives must engage all stakeholders.

The relationship between universal design and AT

The essence of universal design (UD) involves proactively valuing human diversity such that products and environments are "usable by the widest range of people operating in the widest range of situations as is commercially practical" (Vanderheiden, 2000, p. 32). Because some AT is designed with the specific needs of a particular disability or group in mind, there can sometimes be confusion about the relationship between UD and AT and which approach should take priority.

The drivers of change in the AT field

In order to understand the drivers of change over the last 40 years it is necessary to examine three particular pillars of this period: policy, innovative product development and research.

Pillar 1: Policy as a Change Lever

In the United States, and many countries, policy makers have been persuaded to enact legislation encouraging the expansion of AT devices and services based on the compelling evidence from individuals whose lives have been transformed. The historical record (Office of Technology Assessment, 1982) reveals it was case studies and personal testimonies rather than quantifiable research evidence that led to the foundational public investments necessary to expand AT service delivery systems.

Special education has long used federal policy as a change lever (West & Whitby, 2008). Scholars studying the historical evolution of the field of AT will often notice that various eras can be operationalised in relationship to the passage of major federal laws in the United States (Blackhurst, 2005, 1965; Blackhurst & Edyburn, 2000). For example, AT in schools looked very different before, and following, the passage of the Education for All Handicapped Children Act (P.L. 94–142, 1975). Other significant policy milestones in the US include the Technology-Related Assistance Act for Individuals with Disabilities (P.L. 100–407, 1988), the Americans with Disabilities Act (P.L. 101–306, 1990), and the Individuals with Disabilities Education Act (P.L. 105–17, 1997).[3,4,5,6]

Disability advocacy has contributed to increased awareness about accessibility design principles and technical standards. As a result, accessibility solutions in the form of curb cuts, web accessibility standards and accessibility control panels/preferences have scaled. Each of these exemplars illustrates how the evolution of assistive technologies as solutions for individuals (e.g., word prediction, text to speech) could scale into UD applications that provided similar solutions and benefits to mainstream society (e.g., voice assistants). Whereas these developments were not an explicit change strategy, they have served to increase awareness about the value of universal access for people with disabilities (who need such solutions all the time), people with injuries (who need such solutions temporarily as part of the rehabilitation process) and people who value such options as a matter of choice given various circumstances (e.g., shifting the task of reading to listening while driving). These developments illustrate the tension associated with public policy concerning the relationship between AT and UDL. However, it is increasingly common to assess both the use of mainstream technologies and specialised AT when seeking to understand the most efficacious use of technology by individuals with disabilities (Budrionis et al., 2022; Abraham et al., 2021).

The use of policy as a lever of change can also be observed internationally and highlight the importance of understanding a country's particular journey towards inclusive education services and policies (Gronseth & Dalton, 2020; Fineberg et al., 2019; Hemphill et al., 2019). Outside the US, the history of assistive technology is often grounded in post-Internet society (i.e., 2000) and characterised by an infrastructure based on mobile devices such as smartphones (Martiniello et al., 2022). The literature offers valuable insights about the disparate growth and status of AT services around the world, including Africa (Visagie et al., 2017), Australia (Hogan et al., 2023), Brazil (Maximo & Clift, 2015), Cyprus (Wynne, et al., 2016; Mavrou, 2011), Norway (Øien et al., 2016), Sweden (Dahlberg et al., 2014), and the United Kingdom (Chockalingam et al., 2019), as well as regional international efforts (WHO, 2022). Collectively these reports provide insight regarding general trends in AT adoption and implementation. However, the true value of country-specific AT reports is found in their value as case studies of AT as a lever of change in the cultural, educational and political context of a country's inclusive education journey.

Influencing public policy has been an efficient change tactic since it involves lobbying key decision-makers to convince them to advocate for scaling the benefits demonstrated at the individual level to afford the same benefits to the larger population. Some will also argue that policy is a tool for scaling equity and inclusion (Kozleski, 2020). For the foreseeable future, it is not difficult to imagine that we will continue to see legislative and policy initiatives designed to ensure equal access to digital products and services (Chockalingam et al.,

2019). Furthermore, with the perpetual constraints on the public purse, it will be important for AT policy researchers to focus on expanding our understanding of effective policy and practice relative to funding mechanisms (Hogan, et al., 2023; Clayback et al., 2015) and consumer-driven AT acquisition that removes professionals from the procurement process (Manchaiah et al., 2019). Hence, policy research will continue to be an important component of the AT profession as we seek equity and inclusion by capturing the potential of technology for individuals with disabilities.

Pillar 2: Innovative Product Development

Assistive technology solutions have historically been custom engineered for an individual. However, over the past 40 years, the marketplace has developed amazing assistive technology devices that have flipped the paradigm. One comprehensive database, AbleData, documented more than 40,000 AT devices before it ceased operation in 2020. Seeking to address this void, Unified Listing[7] provides a searchable database of accessibility features found in global products. As a result, it is now common practice to begin the AT evaluation process by searching for existing (i.e., off-the-shelf) products that may meet an individual's needs. Modifying existing products and creating custom solutions are still viable solutions but have become much less prevalent as standardised solutions have evolved.

The AT development and commercialisation process has been the subject of considerable research that offers keen insight into the assistive technology industry (Nobrega et al., 2015; Bauer & Flagg, 2010; Lane, 2010, 2008; Leahy & Lane, 2010). Some key lessons learned that have emerged from this literature emphasise the need to involve stakeholders in participatory design (Hobbs et al., 2019; Morris et al., 2019; Jiam et al., 2017; Williamson et al., 2015; Allsop et al., 2011; Francis et al., 2009), the need for iterative product development using agile design methodologies (Edyburn, 2019), and the importance of designing products in accordance with accessibility standards (IMS Global Learning Consortium, 2019).

Despite the current abundance of innovative product solutions, the AT industry faces a number of challenges that could alter its future trajectory. The first challenge is the unresolved relationship between UD and AT and the trade-offs that developers must consider when seeking to secure a share of the market. The expansion of inclusive design principles continues to be applied to mainstream technology products that serve to support diverse users (Kim, 2018) and may ultimately reduce the need for specialised AT for individuals with mild disabilities.

Secondly, perhaps not surprisingly, the economic foundations associated with developing products for small (i.e., niche) markets mean there are very tight margins, which has the effect of fostering dependency on grant funding to sustain research and development work (Bauer & Flagg, 2010; Lane, 2010). Finally, efforts to reach unserved, and underserved, individuals in rural or low-resource environments have fostered innovative approaches for creating and distributing lower-cost AT (Cadeddu et al., 2019; Zahid et al., 2019). However, it remains to be seen whether or not these developments have similar technological and economic disruptive impact as that which occurred in the augmentative and alternative communication (AAC) profession after the introduction of Proloquo2Go.[8] The revolutionary approach of moving an AAC system from large, expensive, dedicated devices to a smartphone app had a significant effect on multiple stakeholders. Users could communicate with the same type of hand-held device as their peers. Families could afford to purchase the app at a fraction of the cost (i.e., less than $200 vs. $7,000 or more). Professionals were no longer gatekeepers in the acquisition process but needed to support a product that they may not be familiar with. Funders were no longer in the business of adjudicating need, and AAC manufacturers of dedicated AAC systems saw their market disappear and some companies went out of business (see Sennott & Bowker, 2009).

Futurists tell us that technological advances will continue at a significant pace because of the innate functions of curiosity, insight and problem-solving (Johnson, 2015; Kelly, 2011). As a result, one can confidently predict that there will continue to be amazing inventions for using technology to enhance human performance, productivity and quality of life. However, we will need to remain diligent in our accessibility advocacy to ensure that new products are accessible and effective for all people. We will also need to continually monitor the public policy investments that may be necessary to support and sustain product development for niche markets like the assistive technology industry.

Pillar 3: Assistive Technology Research

Over the years, the individualised nature of special education and disability services has created a clinical case study orientation to assistive technology research. However, as a result of these advances, the field of assistive technology has benefited from a small number of high-quality research syntheses that inform the profession's knowledge of what works, for whom and under what conditions. While space limitations prevent a comprehensive analysis of the

AT literature, the following key research findings represent examples of the effectiveness of AT that are supported by strong empirical research:

1. AAC interventions are effective for providing voice and communication support for individuals with a variety of disabilities (Morin et al., 2018; Muharib & Alzrayer, 2018; Wren et al., 2018; Ganz et al., 2017; Dunst et al., 2013; Van der Meer & Rispoli, 2010).
2. There are no adverse outcomes associated with providing communication and powered mobility interventions to young children (Romski et al., 2015; Dunst et al., 2013).
3. Assistive technology enables individuals with low vision to effectively access and use information in both learning and employment contexts such that the return-on-investment is clearly demonstrated (Thomas et al., 2015).
4. Assistive technology is effective in the workplace in support of individuals with disabilities in competitive employment (Morash-Macneil et al., 2018).

The field of AT has established silos of research evidence that demonstrate unequivocally that when individuals with disabilities are provided with appropriate AT devices and services, they can reduce the time and frustration of completing some tasks while increasing performance quality. During the past 20 years, the AT research base has grown significantly in terms of the topics we study, the sophistication of our research methodologies and the accumulated evidence about what works. However, for many practitioners, there is an urgent need to make the existing AT knowledge base accessible in ways that inform daily practice.

There is still much more that needs to be understood about the acquisition and use of AT. In recent years, significant advances have been made in operationalising new standards characterising high-quality research (Cooper et al., 2019; Higgins et al., 2019) that have yet to find their way into the AT research community. In addition, there are many noticeable gaps in the literature that need to be addressed to inform AT policy and practice. Examples of such gaps include how to implement a procedure to identify all students who could benefit from AT (similar to how vision and hearing screenings are conducted); the relationship between AT credentials and the quality of practitioner decision-making; the efficacy of various approaches to AT consideration; and longitudinal research designs to understand issues of long-term AT use and device abandonment.

Following a cursory review of the three AT pillars that illustrate how we arrived at this point in time, I will now turn my attention to thinking about the future of AT research; in particular, how the convergence of some existing technologies and data science trends may significantly alter the manner in which AT data are generated, analysed and used.

This is a pivotal juncture as we have seen how the AT profession has been challenged to address outcomes, and now how the future may be impacted by the influence of data scientists, who have little interest in the nuances of assistive technology but will apply their knowledge and skills to the challenges associated with outcomes measurement. The following scenarios are inspired in part by colleagues who have challenged the profession to think about the need for national and international AT outcome measurement systems (Lenker et al., 2021; Scherer et al., 2019).

Future casting: rethinking AT research

There is little evidence to suggest that all people who need, and could benefit from, AT have access to appropriate AT devices and services. Furthermore, there is no evidence to suggest that AT outcome measurement is conducted on a routine basis within existing AT service delivery systems. Without appropriate data collection and research methodologies, the AT profession is at a severe disadvantage when trying to make the argument that AT is an effective public investment that offers a substantial return on investment. As a result, I will argue there is an urgent need to rethink the entire AT enterprise in light of imminent advances in ML and AI. Before delving into the future of AT research, allow me to operationalise some assumptions that I believe foreshadow the anticipated new directions:

1. The future of AT devices may look like an Apple Watch or a Fitbit that is *worn* and/or ubiquitously *mobile* like a smartphone (Wright et al., 2022; Abou et al., 2021; Koumpouros, 2021).
2. AT user profile data will be stored in the cloud and therefore accessible to customise the AT features built into any device (Vanderheiden et al., 2020; Chourasia et al., 2014).
3. AT products will have wireless capabilities that can collect, transmit and analyse location and performance data in real-time similar to how a navigational app (e.g., Google Maps, Waze) works.
4. User data will be collected, transmitted and analysed in a continuous data stream in ways for which the user knowingly grants permission with relevant privacy protections, as well as perhaps in some situations where data are used without the user's knowledge or authorisation (Zuboff, 2019).

5. Consumer-level data analysis tools will enable users to review their personal data any time they like and make decisions, view suggestions or alter settings that enable them to be more successful or effective (Wright et al., 2022; Abou et al., 2021; Koumpouros, 2021).
6. Individual user data will be aggregated into large cloud-based repositories that will offer unprecedented opportunities for artificial intelligence and machine learning applications to mine data in search of patterns and make recommendations for optimisation (Future Today Institute, 2022; Hopcan et al., 2022).

The Gap Between Today and the Future

While I do not have knowledge of, or access to, proprietary cloud-based AT products today, I begin with the proposition that the assumptions outlined earlier have not been currently combined into a single AT product. Yet, it is not hard to imagine how some components could be added to the next generation of AT products. For now I will focus on nine particular technical challenges that I argue will need to be addressed before a new era of AT research is ushered in: (1) connectivity; (2) interoperability; (3) digital workflow; (4) transactional data; (5) frameworks; (6) algorithms; (7) machine learning; (8) artificial intelligence and (9) recommendation engines.

Connectivity

At the present time many AT products do not have connectivity features that allow the transmission of data from the device to a centralised data repository. In the future wireless connectivity will be built into all AT devices. Such features will also support remote firmware and software updates.

Interoperability

Given the nature of the AT industry, few AT products are designed in accordance with interoperability standards to permit devices and systems to share data. In the future AT will need to be designed to conform with interoperability standards to ensure that devices and systems are compatible regardless of the device, location or input method.

Digital workflow

For the most part, current AT assessment systems are paper-based. Similar to the evolution of electronic medical records that moved the medical profession from a paper-based to an electronic-based workflow, the AT profession will need to develop digital case management tools that can talk with other products and systems within the AT ecology.

Transactional data

Given the many types and functions of AT devices, the profession has yet to identify the components of an AT transaction. That is, what data comprise a micro-action of interest and how might data be standardised to capture the end-to-end data associated with this transaction? The field will need to convene an international technical standards workgroup to operationalise approaches to collecting, transmitting and processing AT transactional data – perhaps similar to international credit card processing protocols.

Frameworks

How do we understand components of a comprehensive system of AT devices and services? To manage the complexity, what single-function modules must be developed to perform key tasks within the overall system? Whereas AT professionals may have content knowledge to contribute, it will be essential to collaborate with computer scientists and system engineers to develop the frameworks, logic models and technical standards necessary to collect, store and analyse AT system data.

Algorithms

Collaboration with mathematicians and statisticians will be necessary to develop the algorithms needed to generate computational knowledge. That is, how are constructs like performance or abandonment translated into equations that can be evaluated using computational metrics and inform automated decision-making systems?

Machine learning

AT professionals will need to collaborate with data scientists to explore the application of machine learning to the large data sets generated by AT users. What types of questions do we need to answer? How can we train these new systems using supervised machine learning techniques? How will we ensure that biases are not built into the system?

Artificial intelligence

Whereas machine learning is one component of AI, many other AI applications also have implications for the future of AT research, including: natural language processing, robotics, deep learning and expert systems. Collaboration with AI experts will be necessary to harness the potential of these many forms of advanced technology into a cohesive element of a comprehensive AT system.

Recommendation engines

Given the goal of using AT to improve functional performance, how will human knowledge about performance optimisation be translated into algorithms that generate recommendations? How will machine learning discover new patterns and pathways that humans failed to recognise and improve the quality of AT recommendations to maintain, change or discontinue interventions? How will such recommendations be conveyed and monitored within the digital workflow and individual case management record?

Conclusions: implications for practice

To conclude this chapter, I will outline some suggestions for developing individual and shared research agendas relative to both the short- and intermediate-term future of AT research.

Conceptualising Research

The traditional paradigm has been researcher-generated investigations followed by research-into-practice dissemination (Joyce & Cartwright, 2020). However, the field of AT could benefit from additional practice-inspired collaborative research (Smith & Boger, 2022). Indeed, this is a tenet of participatory research (Koontz et al., 2022) and the necessity of engaging people with disabilities in the design of AT solutions. As a result, I encourage individuals and groups to propose, disseminate and critique proposed research agendas in order to spark conversation, debate and collaboration about the future of AT research. In the words of Reeves and Lin (2020, p. 1991): "The research we have is not the research we need."

Theory

A hallmark of science is theory-driven research; that is, conducting research that supports or refutes a hypothesis given what is known/expected about a phenomenon. Significantly more theoretical work is needed to move the field beyond a simplistic AT theory of change based on buy-use. Existing work by Lenker and colleagues offers an excellent starting point for developing data-driven AT theory (Lenker et al., 2021; Lenker et al., 2012; Lenker et al., 2010; Lenker & Paquet, 2004, 2003).

Impact

For too long the field of AT has relied on *consumer satisfaction* as the outcome of AT use (Ranada & Lidström, 2019) with considerably less attention devoted to measuring performance. As a result, significant work remains to be done to describe the performance of individuals with disabilities when completing routine tasks with, and without, technology tools. Such information will be essential for the development of analytics that can determine who might benefit from AT and what types of performance gains can be expected under varying conditions. Much more work is needed to understand the conditions under which performance is optimised.

Innovation Partnerships

AT developers are incentivised to bring their products to market as soon as possible (Leahy & Lane, 2010; Lane, 2008;). This often means limited research on a product's efficacy. Collaboration between developers and researchers could fill this void by providing initial evidence as a product comes into the marketplace and more comprehensive research as the product is adopted. The availability of large-scale, population-based research data will require that the AT profession become more adept at managing partnerships with a variety of technical disciplines, including experts in artificial intelligence, machine learning, big data, data science, statistical modelling, systems engineering and more.

Data Analytics

Whereas many AT researchers are often stymied by a lack of access to AT data, we are at the precipice of a deluge of data. As a result, there is an urgent need for new tools and analytic frameworks to make sense of the overwhelming volume of data that will be generated as people use their AT. Naturally, data dashboards and data visualisation will become a priority for making sense of basic patterns within the data. However, we will need new theoretical frameworks for ascertaining what it means to use AT effectively in a data-based environment and which variables of AT service delivery systems warrant adjustment.

Privacy

Given the general advances of technology in the consumer market, privacy concerns are likely to be an ongoing challenge to the AT profession. However, there are many examples of how consumer-demand drives the adoption of new technologies despite misgivings about privacy protections (Zuboff, 2019; O'Neil, 2016). This is an area of urgent need for the profession to consider how to implement privacy safeguards while advancing opportunities to use personal data to improve the user experience and product performance.

Transparency

The fundamental nature of unsupervised machine learning (Alloghani et al., 2020) is that scientists do not know how machines are making decisions (O'Neil, 2016). As a result, there is considerable interest in what is known as *ethical AI* (Jobin et al., 2019; Mittelstadt, 2019) and *interpretable AI* (Thampi, 2022) in order to provide a level of transparency and make the decision-making mechanisms accessible to humans. These issues have already been foreshadowed in the context of AT (Goldberg et al., 2022) and are worthy of continued exploration.

In considering my suggestions for developing individual and shared research agendas, I encourage readers to anticipate a future that may be vastly different from the recent past and to engage in the interdisciplinary conversations that will be necessary to guide advances that are already on the horizon and have the potential to dramatically alter the provision and use of assistive technology.

Notes

1   US Code Title 20 Education. https://www.govinfo.gov/content/pkg/USCODE-20 21-title20/pdf/USCODE-2021-title20-chap33-subchapI-sec1401.pdf.
2   The ATOMS Project. https://uwm.edu/r2d2/projects/atoms/.
3   P.L. 94–142, 1975. Education for All Handicapped Children Act. https://www .govinfo.gov/content/pkg/STATUTE-89/pdf/STATUTE-89-Pg773.pdf
4   P.L. 100–407, 1988. Technology-Related Assistance Act for Individuals with Disabilities. https://www.govinfo.gov/content/pkg/STATUTE-102/pdf/STATUTE-1 02-Pg1044.pdf.

5   P.L. 101–306, 1990. The Americans with Disabilities Act.
6   P.L. 105–17, 1997. The Individuals with Disabilities Education Act. https://www
    .govinfo.gov/content/pkg/PLAW-105publ17/pdf/PLAW-105publ17.pdf.
7   Unified Listing. https://ul.gpii.net/.
8   Proloqou2go. https://www.assistiveware.com/products/proloquo2go.

References

Abou, L., Fliflet, A., Hawari, L., Presti, P., Sosnoff, J.J., Mahajan, H.P., Frechette, M.L., & Rice, L.A. (2021). Sensitivity of Apple Watch fall detection feature among wheelchair users. *Assistive Technology, 34*(5), 619–625. https://doi.org/10.1080/10400435.2021.1923087

Abraham, C.H., Boadi-Kusi, B., Morny, E.K.A., & Agyekum, P. (2021). Smartphone usage among people living with severe visual impairment and blindness. *Assistive Technology, 34*(5), 611–618. DOI:10.1080/10400435.2021.1907485

Alloghani, M., Al-Jumeily, D., Mustafina, J., Hussain, A., & Aljaaf, A.J. (2020). A systematic review on supervised and unsupervised machine learning algorithms for data science. In M.W. Very, A. Mohamed, & B.W. Yap (Eds.), *Supervised and Unsupervised Learning for Data Science* (pp. 3–21). Springer. https://doi.org/10.1007/978-3-030-22475-2_1

Allsop, M., Gallagher, J., Holt, R., Bhakta, B., & Wilkie, R. (2011). Involving children in the development of assistive technology devices. *Disability and Rehabilitation: Assistive Technology, 6*(2), 148–156. DOI:10.3109/17483107.2010.510178

Bauer, S.M., & Flagg, J.L. (2010). Technology transfer and technology transfer intermediaries. *Assistive Technology Outcomes and Benefits, 6*(1), 129–150. https://files.eric.ed.gov/fulltext/EJ899223.pdf

Blackhurst, A.E. (2005). Historical perspectives about technology applications for people with disabilities. In D. Edyburn, K. Higgins, & R. Boone (Eds.), *Handbook of Special Education Technology Research and Practice* (pp. 1–27). Knowledge by Design.

Blackhurst, A.E., & Edyburn, D.L. (2000). A brief history of special education technology. *Special Education Technology Practice, 2*(1), 21–35.

Blackhurst, A.E. (1965). Technology in special education – some implications. *Exceptional Children, 31*(9), 449–456 http://mrnoury.weebly.com/uploads/3/7/2/9/37295409/history_of_at.pdf

Budrionis, A., Plikynas, D., Daniušis, P., & Indrulionis, A. (2022). Smartphone-based computer vision travelling aids for blind and visually impaired individuals: A systematic review. *Assistive Technology, 34*(2), 178–194. DOI:10.1080/10400435.2020.1743381

Cadeddu, S.B., Layton, N., Banes, D., & Cadeddu, S. (2019). Frugal innovation and what it offers the assistive technology sector. In N. Layton & J. Borg (Eds.), *Global Perspectives on Assistive Technology: Proceedings of the GReAT Consultation 2019, Volume 2* (pp. 487–502). World Health Organization. https://apps.who.int/iris/handle/10665/330372

Chockalingam, N., Eddison, N., & Healy, A. (2019). Orthotic service provision in the United Kingdom: Does everyone get the same service? In N. Layton & J. Borg (Eds.), *Global Perspectives on Assistive Technology: Proceedings of the GReAT Consultation*

2019, Volume 1 (pp. 515–524). World Health Organization. https://apps.who.int/iris/handle/10665/330371

Chourasia, A., Nordstrom, D., & Vanderheiden, G. (2014). State of the science on the Cloud, accessibility, and the future. *Universal Access in the Information Society, 13*, 483–495. https://doi.org/10.1007/s10209-013-0345-9

Clayback, D., Hostak, R., Leahy, J.A., Minkel, J., Piper, M., Smith, R.O., & Vaarwerk, T. (2015). Standards for assistive technology funding: What are the right criteria. *Assistive Technology Outcomes and Benefits, 9*(1), 40–55.

Cooper, H., Hedges, L.V., & Valentine, J.C. (Eds.) (2019). *The Handbook of Research Synthesis and Meta-analysis.* NY: Russell Sage Foundation.

Dahlberg, R., Blomquist, U.B., Richter, A., & Lampel, A. (2014). The service delivery system for assistive technology in Sweden: Current situation and trends. *Technology and Disability, 26*(4), 191–197. DOI:10.3233/TAD-140416

DeRuyter, F. (1997). The importance of outcome measure for assistive technology service delivery systems. *Technology and Disability, 6*(1–2), 89–104. https://content.iospress.com/articles/technology-and-disability/tad6-1-2-08

Dunst, C.J., Trivette, C.M., Hamby, D.W., & Simkus, A. (2013). Systematic review of studies promoting the use of assistive technology devices by young children with disabilities. *Practical Evaluation Reports, 5*(1), 1–32. https://files.eric.ed.gov/fulltext/ED565254.pdf

Edyburn, D.L. (2019). *App Development for Individuals with Disabilities: Insights for Developers and Entrepreneurs.* Knowledge by Design.

Edyburn, D.L. (2013). Critical issues in advancing the special education technology evidence-base. *Exceptional Children, 80*(1), 7–24. https://journals.sagepub.com/doi/10.1177/001440291308000107

Edyburn, D.L. (2003). Rethinking assistive technology. *Special Education Technology Practice, 5*(4), 16–22. https://doi.org/10.1177/016264340401900106

Edyburn, D.L. (2002). Measuring assistive technology outcomes: Key concepts. *Journal of Special Education Technology, 18*(1), 53–55. https://doi.org/10.1177/016264340301800107

Fineberg, A.E., Savage, M., Austinc, V., Boiten, S., Droop, J., Allen, M., Heydt, P., Sondergaard, D., & Mitra, G. (2019). ATscale – Establishing a cross-sector partnership to increase access to assistive technology. In N. Layton & J. Borg (Eds.), *Global Perspectives on Assistive Technology: Proceedings of the GReAT Consultation 2019*, Volume 2 (pp. 428–439). World Health Organization. https://apps.who.int/iris/handle/10665/330372

Francis, P., Mellor, D., & Firth, L. (2009). Techniques and recommendations for the inclusion of users with autism in the design of assistive technologies. *Assistive Technology, 21*(2), 57–68. https://doi.org/10.1080/10400430902945561

Future Today Institute (2022). Tech Trends. https://futuretodayinstitute.com/trends/

Ganz, J.B., Morin, K.L., Foster, M.J., Vannest, K.J., Genç Tosun, D., Gregori, E.V., & Gerow, S.L. (2017). High-technology augmentative and alternative communication for individuals with intellectual and developmental disabilities and complex communication needs: A meta-analysis. *Augmentative and Alternative Communication, 33*(4), 224–238. https://doi.org/10.1080/07434618.2017.1373855

Goldberg, M., Karimi, H., Jordan, J.B., & Lazar, J. (2022). Are accessible software accountable? A commentary. *Assistive Technology, 34*(1), 61–63. https://doi.org/10.1080/10400435.2021.2024627

Gronseth, S.L., & Dalton, E.M. (2020). *Universal Access through Inclusive Instructional Design: International Perspectives on UDL.* Routledge.

Hemphill, C., Layton, N., Banes, D., Long, S., & Hemphill, C. (2019). Evaluating the economics of assistive technology provision. In N. Layton & J. Borg (Eds.), *Global Perspectives on Assistive Technology: Proceedings of the GReAT Consultation 2019, Volume 1* (pp. 248–268). World Health Organization. https:// apps .who .int/ iris/ handle/10665/330372

Higgins, J.P., Thomas, J., Chandler, J., Compton, M., Li, T, Page, M.J., & Welch, V.A. (Eds.) (2019). *Cochrane Handbook for Systematic Reviews of Interventions* (2nd ed.). John Wiley & Sons.

Hobbs, D., Walker, S., Layton, N., & Hobbs, D. (2019). Appropriate assistive technology co-design: From problem identification through to device commercialisation. In N. Layton & J. Borg (Eds.), *Global Perspectives on Assistive Technology: Proceedings of the GReAT Consultation 2019, Volume 2* (pp. 342–358). World Health Organization. https://apps.who.int/iris/handle/10665/330372

Hogan, C., Gustafsson, L., Di Tommaso, A., Hodson, T., Bissett, M., & Shirota, C. (2023). Establishing the normative and comparative needs of assistive technology provision in Queensland from the agency and funding scheme perspective. *Brain Impairment*, 1–15. DOI:10.1017/BrImp.2023.10

Hopcan, S., Polat, E., Ozturk, M.E., & Ozturk, L. (2022). Artificial intelligence in special education: A systematic review. *Interactive Learning Environments*. https://doi.org/10.1080/10494820.2022.2067186

IMS Global Learning Consortium (2019). IMS Global AccessforAll (AfA) Primer. Retrieved from http://www.imsglobal.org/activity/accessibility

Jiam, N.T., Hoon, A.H., Hostetter, C.F., & Khare, M.M. (2017). IIAM (important information about me): A patient portability profile app for adults, children and families with neurodevelopmental disabilities. *Disability and Rehabilitation: Assistive Technology, 12*(6), 599–604. DOI:10.1080/17483107.2016.1198435

Jobin, A., Ienca, M., & Vayena, E. (2019). The global landscape of AI ethics guidelines. *Nature Machine Intelligence, 1*(9), 389–399. https:// doi .org/ 10 .1038/ s42256 -019-0088-2

Johnson, S. (2015). *How We Got to Now: Six Innovations That Made the Modern World.* Riverhead Books.

Joyce, K.E., & Cartwright, N. (2020). Bridging the gap between research and practice: Predicting what will work locally. *American Educational Research Journal, 57*(3), 1045–1082. https://doi.org/10.3102/0002831219866687

Kelly, K. (2011). *What Technology Wants.* Penguin.

Kim, H.N. (2018). User experience of mainstream and assistive technologies for people with visual impairments. *Technology and Disability, 30*(3), 127–133. DOI:10.3233/TAD-180191

Koontz, A., Duvall, J., Johnson, R., Reissman, T., & Smith, E. (2022). 'Nothing about us without us': Engaging AT users in AT research. *Assistive Technology, 34*(5), 499–500. https://doi.org/10.1080/10400435.2022.2117524

Koumpouros, Y. (2021). An 'all-in-one' wearable application for assisting children with Autism Spectrum Disorder. *Technology and Disability, 33*(1), 65–75. DOI:10.3233/TAD-200291

Kozleski, E.B. (2020). Disrupting what passes as inclusive education: Predicating educational equity on schools designed for all. *Educational Forum, 84*(4), 340–355. https://doi.org/10.1080/00131725.2020.1801047

Lane, J.P. (2010). State of the science in technology transfer: At the confluence of academic research and business development – Merging technology transfer with knowledge translation to deliver value. *Assistive Technology Outcomes and Benefits,* 6(1), 1–38. https://files.eric.ed.gov/fulltext/EJ899218.pdf

Lane, J.P. (2008). Delivering on the D in R&D: Recommendations for increasing transfer outcomes from development projects. *Assistive Technology Outcomes and Benefits,* 5(1), 1–60.

Leahy, J.A., & Lane, J.P. (2010). Knowledge from research and practice on the barriers and carriers to successful technology transfer for assistive technology devices. *Assistive Technology Outcomes and Benefits,* 6(1), 73–86. https:// files .eric .ed .gov/ fulltext/EJ899220.pdf

Lenker, J.A., Koester, H.H., & Smith, R.O. (2021). Toward a national system of assistive technology outcomes measurement. *Assistive Technology, 33*(1), 1–8. DOI:10.1080/ 10400435.2019.1567620

Lenker, J.A., Shoemaker, L.L., Fuhrer, M.J., Jutai, J.W., Demers, L., Tan, C.H., & DeRuyter, F. (2012). Classification of assistive technology services: Implications for outcomes research. *Technology and Disability, 24*(1), 59–70. DOI: 10.3233/ TAD-2012-0334

Lenker, J.A., Fuher, M.J., Jutai, J.W., Demers, L., Scherer, M.J., & DeRuyter, F. (2010). Treatment theory, intervention specification, and treatment fidelity in assistive technology outcome research. *Assistive Technology, 22*(3), 129–138. DOI:10.1080/10400430903519910

Lenker, J.A., & Paquet, V.L. (2004). A new conceptual model for assistive technology outcomes and research. *Assistive Technology, 16*(1), 1–10. DOI:10.1080/10400435.2 004.10132069

Lenker, J.A., & Paquet, V.L. (2003). A review of conceptual models for assistive technology outcomes research and practice. *Assistive Technology, 15*(1), 1–15. DOI:10.1 080/10400435.2003.10131885

Manchaiah, V., Amlani, A.M., Bricker, C.M., Whitfield, C.T., & Ratinaud, P. (2019). Benefits and shortcomings of direct-to-consumer hearing devices: Analysis of large secondary data generated from Amazon customer reviews. *Journal of Speech, Language, and Hearing Research, 62*(5), 1506–1516. DOI:10.1044/2018_JSLHR-H-18-0370

Martiniello, N., Eisenbarth, W., Lehane, C., Johnson, A., & Wittich, W. (2022). Exploring the use of smartphones and tablets among people with visual impairments: Are mainstream devices replacing the use of traditional visual aids? *Assistive Technology, 34*(1), 34–45. DOI:10.1080/10400435.2019.1682084

Mavrou, K. (2011). Assistive technology as an emerging policy and practice: Processes, challenges and future directions. *Technology and Disability, 23*(1), 41–52. DOI:10.3233/TAD-2011-0311

Maximo, T., & Clift, L. (2015). Assessing service delivery systems for assistive technology in Brazil using HEART study quality indicators. *Technology and Disability, 27*(4), 161–170. DOI:10.3233/TAD-160438

Mittelstadt, B. (2019). Principles alone cannot guarantee ethical AI. *Nature Machine Intelligence, 1*(11), 501–507. https://doi.org/10.1038/s42256-019-0114-4

Morash-Macneil, V., Johnson, F., & Ryan, J.B. (2018). A systematic review of assistive technology for individuals with intellectual disability in the workplace. *Journal of Special Education Technology, 33*(1), 15–26. https:// doi .org/ 10 .1177/ 0162643417729166

Morin, K.L., Ganz, J.B., Gregori, E.V., Foster, M.J., Gerow, S.L., Genç-Tosun, D., & Hong, E. R. (2018). A systematic quality review of high-tech AAC interventions as an evidence-based practice. *Augmentative and Alternative Communication, 34*(2), 104–117. https://doi.org/10.1080/07434618.2018.1458900

Morris, J., Thompson, N., Lippincott, B., & Lawrence, M. (2019). Accessibility user research collective: Engaging consumers in ongoing technology evaluation. *Assistive Technology Outcomes and Benefits,* 13, 38–56. https:// www .atia .org/ wp -content/ uploads/2019/10/ATOB-V13-FINAL_Morris.pdf

Muharib, R., & Alzrayer, N.M. (2018). The use of high-tech speech-generating devices as an evidence-based practice for children with autism spectrum disorders: A meta-analysis. Review. *Journal of Autism and Developmental Disorders, 5*(1), 43–57. https://doi.org/10.1007/s40489-017-0122-4

Nobrega, A.R., Lane, J.P., Flagg, J.L., Stone, V.I., Lockett, M., Oddo, C., Leahy, C., Usiak, J.A & Douglas, D. (2015). Assessing the roles of national organizations in research-based knowledge creation, engagement and translation: Comparative results across three assistive technology application areas. *Assistive Technology Outcomes and Benefits, 9*(1), 54–97.

Office of Technology Assessment (1982). *Technology and Handicapped People.* U.S. Government Printing Office.

Øien, I., Fallang, B., & Østensjø, S. (2016). Everyday use of assistive technology devices in school settings. *Disability and Rehabilitation: Assistive Technology, 11*(8), 630–635. DOI:10.3109/17483107.2014.1001449

O'Neil, C. (2016). *Weapons of Math Destruction.* Broadway Books.

Ranada, A.L. & Lidström, H. (2019). Satisfaction with assistive technology device in relation to the service delivery process – A systematic review. *Assistive Technology, 31*(2), 82–97. DOI:10.1080/10400435.2017.1367737

Reeves, T.C., & Lin, L. (2020). The research we have is not the research we need. *Educational Technology Research and Development, 68,* 1991–2001. https://doi.org/ 10.1007/s11423-020-09811-3

Romski, M., Sevcik, R.A., Barton-Hulsey, A., & Whitmore, A.S. (2015). Early intervention and AAC: What a difference 30 years makes. *Augmentative and Alternative Communication, 31*(3), 181–202. DOI:10.3109/07434618.2015.1064163

Rust, K.L., & Smith, R.O. (2006). Perspectives of outcome data from assistive technology developers. *Assistive Technology Outcomes and Benefits, 3*(1), 34–52. https://files .eric.ed.gov/fulltext/EJ902504.pdf

Scherer, M., Smith, R.O., & Layton, N. (2019). Committing to assistive technology outcomes and synthesizing practice, research and policy. In N. Layton & J. Borg (Eds.), *Global Perspectives on Assistive Technology: Proceedings of the GReAT Consultation 2019, Volume 1* (pp. 196–217). World Health Organization. https:// apps .who .int/ iris/handle/10665/330372

Sennott, S., & Bowker, A. (2009). Autism, AAC, and Proloquo2go. *Perspectives on Augmentative and Alternative Communication, 18*(4), 137–145. https:// doi.org/ 10 .1044/aac18.4.137

Smith, E.M., & Boger, J. (2022). Better together: Promoting interdisciplinary research in assistive technology. *Assistive Technology, 34*(1), 1–1. https:// doi .org/ 10 .1080/ 10400435.2022.2047397

Thampi, A. (2022). *Interpretable AI.* Manning Publications.

Thomas, R., Barker, L., Rubin, G., & Dahlmann Noor, A. (2015). Assistive technology for children and young people with low vision. *Cochrane Database of Systematic Reviews, 6,* Art. No.: CD011350. DOI:10.1002/14651858.CD011350.pub2

U.S. Department of Education (2006 & Supp. V. 2011). Individuals With Disabilities Education Act, 20 U.S.C. §§ 1400 et seq.

Van der Meer, L.A., & Rispoli, M. (2010). Communication interventions involving speech-generating devices for children with autism: A review of the literature. *Developmental Neurorehabilitation, 13*(4), 294–306. https://doi.org/10.3109/17518421003671494

Vanderheiden, G.C., Lazar, J., Jordan, J.B., Ding, Y., & Wood, R.E. (2020). Morphic: Auto-personalization on a global scale. *Proceedings of the 2020 CHI Conference on Human Factors in Computing Systems* (pp. 1–12). ACM. https://doi.org/10.1145/3313831.3376204

Vanderheiden, G.C. (2000). Fundamental principles and priority setting for universal usability. *Proceedings of the 2000 Conference on Universal Usability* (pp. 32–37). ACM. http://www.acm.org/pubs/articles/proceedings/chi/355460/p32-vanderheiden/p32-vanderheiden.pdf

Visagie, S., Eide, A.H., Mannan, H., Schneider, M., Swartz, L., Mji, G., Munthall, A., Khogali, M., Rooy, G.V., & MacLachlan, M. (2017). A description of assistive technology sources, services and outcomes of use in a number of African settings. *Disability and Rehabilitation: Assistive Technology, 12*(7), 705–712. https://doi.org/10.1080/17483107.2016.1244293

West, J.E., & Whitby, P.J. (2008). Federal policy and education of students with disabilities: Progress and the path forward. *Focus on Exceptional Children, 41*(3), 1–16.

Williamson, T., Kenney, L., Barker, A.T., Cooper, G., Good, T., Healey, J., Heller, B., Howard, D., Mathews, M., Prenton, S., Ryan, J., & Smith, C. (2015). Enhancing public involvement in assistive technology design research. *Disability and Rehabilitation: Assistive Technology, 10*(3), 258–265. https://doi.org/10.3109/17483107.2014.908247

World Health Organization (2022). *Strategic Action Framework to Improve Access to Assistive Technology in the Eastern Mediterranean Region.* https://apps.who.int/iris/bitstream/handle/10665/352488/9789290226604-eng.pdf

Wren, Y., Harding, S., Goldbart, J., & Roulstone, S. (2018). A systematic review and classification of interventions for speech-sound disorder in preschool children. *International Journal of Language & Communication Disorders, 53*(3), 446–467. https://doi.org/10.1111/1460-6984.12371

Wright, R.E., McMahon, D.D., Cihak, D.F., & Hirschfelder, K. (2022). Smartwatch executive function supports for students with ID and ASD. *Journal of Special Education Technology, 37*(1), 63–73. https://doi.org/10.1177/0162643420950027

Wynne, R., McAnaney, D., MacKeogh, T., Stapleton, P., Delaney, S., Dowling, N., & Jeffares, I. (2016). *Assistive Technology/Equipment in Supporting the Education of Children with Special Educational Needs – What Works Best? Research Report Number 22.* National Council for Special Education. http://ncse.ie/wp-content/uploads/2016/07/NCSE-Assistive-Technology-Research-Report-No22.pdf

Zahid, A., Krumins, V., & De Witte, L. (2019). The development of innovation sharing platforms for low cost and do-it-yourself assistive technology in low and middle-income countries. In N. Layton & J. Borg (Eds.), *Global Perspectives on Assistive Technology: Proceedings of the GReAT Consultation 2019, Volume 2* (pp. 359–376). World Health Organization. https://apps.who.int/iris/handle/10665/330372

Zuboff, S. (2019). *The Age of Surveillance Capitalism: The Fight for a Human Future at the New Frontier of Power.* Profile Books.

8. How the professional training of Assistive Technologists can inform a future research agenda

Rohan Slaughter, Annalu Waller and Tom Griffiths

Introduction

This chapter was written in the latter part of 2022 and in the first quarter of 2023. At the time of writing, the MSc Educational AT (MSc EduAT) at the University of Dundee had been running for just over two years, with the first cohort about to graduate. The third cohort had completed their first core modules and the fourth cohort was being actively recruited. The course is now an established part of the assistive technology (AT) training landscape in the United Kingdom.

People tend to 'fall into' AT from various backgrounds, in part due to the lack of a formal route into AT roles, along with the lack of a clear definition of the AT role. There have been previous attempts to create a structured AT-focused postgraduate course, and these courses are no longer offered (see, for example, Seale & Turner-Smith, 2001 who describe the Kings College, London, Masters in AT). However, previous efforts have concentrated on particular sectors or aspects of AT and focused on AT in its broadest definition; including technology to support people with a range of disabilities and health conditions, as well as meet the needs of an ageing population, having an emphasis on health or age, as well as disability. In the United States, RESNA (Rehabilitation Engineering and AT Society of North America) has two qualification routes which are offered to AT professionals and specifically to rehabilitation engineers and seating and mobility specialists.[1] In Europe there have been a number of efforts to support the teaching of AT (Whitney et al., 2011). Again, some of these courses are focused on rehabilitation engineering and others support training in universal design or accessibility. As far as the authors are aware, there has not previously been a strategically informed, transdisciplinary approach to professionalising the Assistive Technologist role through the development of a qualification which is underpinned by research and a strong commitment to including and valuing disabled people's experiences.

Integrating the views of MSc EduAT students is essential, and the programme team must ensure that students are supported to collect the views of the people that they work with, who are the users of the AT systems. The members of the various groups within the User Centre at the University of Dundee also inform the approach and have supported programme developments. The User Centre groups are a unique feature of the discipline of Computing at the University of Dundee and ensure that research and teaching projects across the University are scrutinised by people who are expert users of AT.[2] For example, members of the user centre who are expert users of AT provide feedback to second-year students presenting early-stage or planned development of their dissertation projects at the EduAT on-campus teaching and conference week.

Within the EduAT programme team there is a strong commitment to active collaboration with colleagues from across the AT sector, without which any efforts to professionalise the AT role are unlikely to succeed. To this end the EduAT programme team have taken opportunities to support and collaborate with colleagues from a range of organisations in a collegiate and open way.

The university is an active associate member of APPGAT (All-Party Parliamentary Group for AT), which has its secretariat with Policy Connect, a non-partisan think tank.[3] All-party parliamentary groups are informal cross-party groups. While they do not have official status within parliament, they are useful to bring together policy makers, and experts from a variety of organisations, including academia, commercial companies and charities to support evidence-based policy making. The programme team are actively supporting the inclusive efforts of the APPGAT to develop effective, and evidence-based, AT policy proposals.

The programme team have the support of an advisory group. This group includes academics from other higher education organisations, service delivery professionals from the specialist and mainstream education sectors, disabled people in a variety of national policy support roles and professionals working in sector support bodies. The MSc EduAT advisory group act as 'critical friends' to the programme team to support curriculum design and delivery. The terms of reference for this group were born out of the MSc EduAT development process and enable the group to both support and challenge the programme team in a way that enhances the course delivery.

The authors recognise that the professionalisation of an emerging professional role cannot be done by the development of a single new course, or indeed by a single entity such as a university. There are various ways of supporting the professionalisation of the AT role. It is not thought likely that the government would legislate to create a protected title, as the sector is small. The perceived risks and benefits of such a time-intensive route mean it is thought to be unlikely for professionalisation to be supported in this way. It may, however, be possible to support the creation of a professional body for Assistive Technologists that could encourage the professionalisation of the role, develop CPD standards for both formative and in-service training and development requirements and establish itself as a recognised authority on AT in the UK. Recent research commissioned by the UK government's Department of Education (Edyburn, 2020) made five recommendations that align with aspects of our approach:

1. Develop personnel preparation pathways that provide general AT knowledge
2. Develop personnel preparation pathways that develop specialised AT knowledge
3. Establish AT teams
4. Standardise AT evaluation procedures and protocols
5. Connect AT devices, AT services with AT outcomes

The development of courses that can provide training for staff in both general AT as well as specialised AT support is part of the EduAT approach outlined in this chapter. We recognise the need to establish AT teams and to develop and standardise 'AT Evaluation Procedures and Protocols', and we concur that there is a need to ensure that the outcomes of AT services are recorded and further researched to evidence the impact of the service provided. In summary we propose that raising the quality of AT service delivery through professionalising the field is important. It is overdue for this emergent profession to ensure quality and continuous improvement of AT assessment, and provisioning and ongoing support for AT delivery by implementing formalised quality assurance and quality improvement mechanisms. These mechanisms do require definition and development and are seen as a vital part of the efforts to professionalise the Assistive Technologist role.

This chapter explores the need and drivers behind calls to professionalise the AT role. It will include an overview of why the programme team developed the MSc EduAT, including a summary of what we have learned after two years of developing and running the programme. The chapter considers that AT is in some ways in a 'golden age', with a broader range of accessible technology available than ever before as well as technology being more affordable for everyone. We consider that not all members of the AT workforce need a Masters level qualification, with instead a range of courses provided at multiple levels, underpinned by a development framework.

The chapter closes by defining a research agenda that has been informed by the development of the MSc EduAT and the experience and input of the staff team and the students who have pioneered this new course with the programme team.

Why professionalise the AT role?

In exploring justifications for the call to professionalise the AT role, we will first define AT and the AT role. We will then examine drivers for professionalisation and consider how the role integrates with other professions.

Defining AT and the Assistive Technologist Role

There currently exists no agreed definition of the AT role, with local definitions being highly dependent on the context in which the role holders work. Assistive Technologists are found in education-, health- and social care-focused roles. This variance is due in part to the fact that AT itself has many context-dependent definitions; the World Health Organization (WHO, 2023) definition is very broad, as it includes aids to daily living, mobility aids and other technologies that are widely available in an advanced healthcare economy such as the United Kingdom. A tighter definition to specifically address electronic AT may be helpful here, in part to separate the professional development programme of the MSc EduAT from existing pathways for rehabilitation engineers or healthcare and clinical scientists (for example the Rehabilitation Engineering and Assistive Technologies MSc at UCL).[4]

With a view to support the development of the AT role, members of the programme team worked with colleagues from The TechAbility Service at Natspec (National Specialist Colleges Association[5]) to develop a dedicated entry in the ESCO (European Standards, Competencies and Occupations) database for the Assistive Technologist role:

> Assistive Technologists work to improve access to learning or/and improving independence and participation for individuals with disabilities. They do this through learner support and staff support with activities such as assessments, training and

guidance. Assistive Technologists have a good understanding of learners' needs and a wide technology knowledge relevant to learning, living or work context. The role requires knowledge of AT hardware and software such as text to speech, prediction, dictation, vision and physical access tools. (ESCO, 2022)

Defining the role of an Assistive Technologist who operates in contexts such as education, social care, the third sector and beyond is possible in part by saying what it is not. The motivation for the selection of 'Educational AT' (EduAT) for the name of the degree programme was to ensure some differentiation from existing approaches and training routes. The key point to emphasise is that the EduAT approach is not medically derived but instead reflects a more socially inclusive approach. The closest professional grouping is teaching or education, reflecting the strong 'train the trainer' emphasis placed on the EduAT definition of the AT role. Note that those who undertake the EduAT role do not have to be working in education organisations; indeed students are also drawn from various third sector, private practice, therapy, health and social care organisations. The EduAT approach is a fusion of the knowledge, skills and attributes of education and teaching roles, health or therapy roles and computing, IT and AT roles. It is by nature a transdisciplinary role; the EduAT does not replace any existing role, but rather complements and supports colleagues in existing roles.

Drivers for Professionalisation

Drivers for professionalisation of the AT role began with requests for AT training or courses to help develop colleagues from across the education sector and beyond. The Jisc (Joint Information Services Committee)-funded Dart Project (Slaughter & Mobbs, 2015) identified a need (and demand) for training and support for AT professionals in further education organisations and beyond. The Dart Project research (Maudslay, 2015) identified that, where there were dedicated AT roles, organisations benefited from significant improvements to AT outcomes for their students. These themes have been further explored and updated in the dissertation projects of EduAT students, some of which are planned to be published during 2023.

There is a growing trend for head teachers, college leaders and others, having identified the need for an AT specialist role, to attempt to recruit to dedicated Assistive Technologist roles, with varying degrees of success. The Dart Project role profile and person specification for the AT role has been replicated in a range of organisations. As these documents were widely shared, many of the Assistive Technologists employed in UK-based mainstream and specialist education organisations today can trace their role profile or person specifications development back to these template documents. However, even when organisations chose to implement or develop such dedicated AT roles it continued to be difficult to recruit. In some cases, there was a lack of assurance or confidence that candidates were high-quality or had a broad enough experience of supporting AT. This was in part perceived to be due to the lack of a protected title. Because anyone can claim the title, some leaders concluded that it would be impossible to tell if applicants were up to the task, resulting in a preference to identify a member of their existing team to develop into the AT role. This experience is directly informed by consultancy work undertaken by the EduAT programme team.

This 'grow your own' approach does have merit. Existing staff members understand their employing organisations and the client group of learners or people who use the service better than someone joining the organisation. However, the lack of an obvious training and development route into the AT role was still a barrier to be overcome. The Dart Projects (2010 to 2015) sought to address this lack of a formal AT training route by developing the 'Dart Curriculum', which aimed to index the few available courses that were offered by academic organisations, AT software or hardware companies, or by people in private practice. This signposting was also augmented by a series of workshops that were offered in different parts of the country, notably at Queen Alexandra College in Birmingham and at the College Development Network Headquarters in Stirling, Scotland.[6,7] Workshop design and content were informed by the first of two research projects undertaken as part of the project.

Part of the reason for the success of the Dart Projects was that training and development was offered to people who were already working to support AT, and who needed to develop their knowledge, skills and understanding. There was, and to some extent still is, a challenge in defining an expected level of AT practice. The Natspec TechAbility Standards (Natspec, 2023) were defined to support AT service improvement in specialist colleges and beyond. Defining what good AT provision looks like continues to be a challenge and is being improved by initiatives to support the understanding of regulators. There are examples where Ofsted (The Office for Standards in Education, Children's Services and Skills) has highlighted the AT role and the impact of assistive technologies such as the assistive technology and AAC (augmentative alternative communication) good practice example from Royal College Manchester (Ofsted, 2015). There are also examples where a single line in an Ofsted report calling for improved AT provision has resulted in the creation of AT posts such as the Assistive Technologist.

The requirement to ensure high-quality service delivery continues to be a strong driver for professionalising the AT role. All education, health and social care organisations are accountable to various regulators such as CQC (Care Quality Commission) and Ofsted in England and the equivalent bodies in the other devolved nations that make up the UK.[8,9] Demonstrating the impact of the AT role and accounting for this through curriculum recording systems is essential to many organisations who have to provide justification for how their publicly funded budgets are spent.

How Does the Assistive Technologist Role Integrate with Other Professions?

The perceptions of other professionals involved in the assessment, provisioning and ongoing support of AT may be unfavourable in some cases, with other professionals identifying the Assistive Technologist role as a 'technician grade' post. In some cases, this is due to the misguided view that this role will impinge on their own professional practice. In this way the work of the EduAT may be deprecated or even ignored by other professional colleagues. The authors have direct experience of this happening in different contexts. In addition, some EduAT students have reported such difficulties when attempting to implement methods of inter- or transdisciplinary working in their employing organisations. In the worst examples, Assistive Technologists have chosen to leave organisations where their skills are not valued or respected. When this does happen it may highlight succession planning concerns as it is often very difficult to replace such specialist staff.

The essential skills, competencies and knowledge as well as the optional skills, competencies and knowledge that make up an EduAT can be seen in the ESCO database entry for the Assistive Technologist, which shows the elements that are required for this role (ESCO, 2022). It should be noted that the EduAT competency framework used in the MSc EduAT programme greatly expands the skills, competences and knowledge beyond the ESCO definition of the role. The reason for this is to cover the broad range of contexts that the role operates within and to support students to consider which parts of the EduAT competency framework apply to their role, and therefore should form part of their learning journey. Most people undertaking EduAT already have a professional context: this could be teaching-, therapy- or technologically-based. As has been identified, the Assistive Technologist is a transdisciplinary role that integrates knowledge skills and understanding from a range of other roles, and these are included within the EduAT competency framework. Development of effective working methodologies to enable collaborative working and integration with other professionals is an important factor that is included in the MSc EduAT programme.

It is important to focus on ongoing professional development for the role, and this is why the EduAT competency framework emphasises the need for professional standards as part of an ethical framework for practice. The EduAT competency framework points to a range of existing skills and knowledge from other professions, and this range matches the available elective modules within MSc EduAT. Students are encouraged to use the elective modules to address their learning opportunities.

Overview of MSc EduAT at the University of Dundee

The design of any new MSc programme is a significant undertaking. This has been even more challenging in the case of the EduAT degree, due to the small pool of potential teaching staff. It took a year from first advertisement to the appointment of a second lecturer, further illustrating the difficulty in developing a new approach to training Assistive Technologists. At the time of writing, there are over 30 students or graduates who have completed, or who are currently enrolled on, the MSc EduAT. This represents a significant increase in the number of people in the UK who are trained at a postgraduate level in AT-related areas. Indeed the fourth cohort for MSc EduAT due to start in January 2024 may be the largest cohort yet.

The Genesis of the MSc EduAT

The Dart Project (Maudslay, 2015) was funded by LSIS (Learning and Skills Improvement Service) and Jisc 2010–2015. As part of Dart, a curriculum was developed to train Assistive Technologists. The Dart curriculum has inspired the approach taken in MSc EduAT and has been expanded upon considerably. In 2014 attempts were made to create the MSc; these did not materialise until early 2019 when a small group gathered to consider core module scope and structure. By the end of 2019, the first author had drafted the programme specification and the specification for the core modules. During 2020 the core modules and the programme specification were scrutinised internally and approved mid-2020.

The first author was appointed as senior lecturer in late 2020 to begin the development and delivery of the MSc EduAT. The programme development has benefited greatly from the advice and encouragement of expert colleagues interested in AT from across the education sector and academia who formed the MSc EduAT advisory group.

The MSc EduAT Curriculum

The MSc EduAT (University of Dundee, 2023) has six core modules which collectively amount to 100 credits:

1. The Educational Assistive Technologist
2. Introduction to AT systems
3. Mainstream and specialist AT
4. Assessment for AT
5. AT in educational programmes
6. AT partner relationships

In addition students select 40 elective credits and choose a 40-credit project dissertation. The 100 core, 40 elective and 40 project dissertation credits make up the 180 credits required for an MSc award (see Figure 8.1).

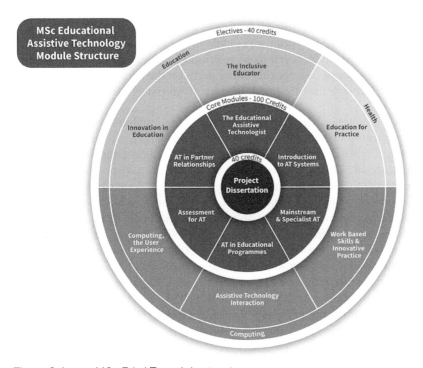

Figure 8.1   MSc EduAT module structure

The first module uses a guided tutorial approach to guide students to undertake a supportive gap analysis using the EduAT competency framework. This is also the focus of the first assessment that is undertaken by students; a reflective piece that encourages students to 'argue out with themselves' where they can get the best value out of their elective module choices. Based on identifying gaps in their knowledge, the student with support from the programme team suggests elective modules from education, computing or IT and health or therapy to address the learning opportunities that have been identified as requiring development in the EduAT competency framework.

Module one establishes the nature of the role, how it can change for different contexts and shares context and background information of relevance. The module also establishes a common understanding of the EduAT role and defines 'The EduAT method'. Modules two and three cover the broad spectrum of available electronic AT and accessories, inclusive of hardware, software, integrated accessibility affordances, mounting and positioning equipment, etc. Module four provides the theoretical basis for the assessment of AT and includes a range of different examples of formal AT assessments, including assessment for AAC, DSA (disabled students allowance) and EAT (electronic AT). Module five provides students with the tools to embed AT within taught programmes and the final core module covers the professional context of the role and how students can make referrals to various parts of the education, health and social care systems. More detail on the core and elective modules can be found on the MSc EduAT website (University of Dundee, 2023).

There are three 'Computing'-focused elective modules. *AT Interaction* is a reimaging of human computer interaction (HCI), with examples drawn from AT. Students are introduced to usability engineering, learning how to evaluate and design user interfaces, with a view to taking an evidence-based approach to influencing and assessing the effective design of AT. *Work-based Skills and Innovative Practice*, which requires the student to design their own learning outcomes, providing an opportunity to research an area of practice of interest to them with academic support. This allows students to engage in a range of learning including work placements, literature reviews and employment-specific innovations such as the introduction of a new way of working. *An Introduction to User Experience* (UX) equips students with skills and approaches to designing systems which are more intuitive using design patterns and design principles. An understanding of this theory is crucial to ensure successful design within a wider context.

There are two 'Education'-focused elective modules. *The Inclusive Educator* provides an overview of inclusion models and specialist education and puts this into context using current legislation and policy. *Innovation in Education* provides background on the drivers for educational reform and supports students to undertake an education innovation project within their workplace. A *Health-led Education for Practice* module is also available, which supports people with a health background to develop their knowledge and skills in education.

We are exploring adding additional elective modules as part of a multi-pathway future evolution of MSc EduAT to enable students to select a pathway best suited to their employment, or future career development pathway. This would enable students to select highly-specialist content such as AAC or complex access if these were focus areas within their employment context.

The course is 'blended', with the majority of delivery online as students are based UK-wide. Most students work full time and undertake MSc EduAT coursework within their working contexts. There are no exams, all assessment is via coursework. Coursework is designed so that students use work they are conducting in their employment as a basis for their academic work. This makes the assessment relevant to students' working contexts and more achievable overall, while working full time. One on-campus teaching and conference week is undertaken per year of part-time study. Entry requirements have been kept as flexible as possible to support a diverse range of students to join the course.

The course is 'profession-agnostic' and is aimed at anyone who wishes to become an Educational Assistive Technologist (EduAT). Students could be teachers or teaching assistants; therapists or therapy assistants/technicians; technologists from a variety of backgrounds; engineers; scientists or technicians. Most students have prior AT experience and are employed in a suitable AT environment. These environments include education, social care or third sector organisations and in a role that typically requires the post holder to support the use of AT. Where a student is not employed in a suitable context work placements will be identified; this is notably important for students who wish to undertake the course full time over two years.

What has been learned?

The students who are taking MSc EduAT are employed in a range of different organisations: sector membership bodies; specialist and mainstream schools and colleges; third sector (charity) and care organisations; higher education institutions; private AT or AAC practice and therapy services; local authorities (advisory teachers or electronic AT specialists); and the National Health Service (NHS). The first cohort includes students working in 'AT - mature' organisations. This is to be expected as students in the cohort joined to develop their skills, address learning opportunities and validate their existing skills and knowledge. The second and third cohorts are drawn from a more diverse range of organisations. International students have been made offers for 2024 entry and the EduAT team are developing AT placement opportunities with partner organisations in many of the types of organisations from which our part-time students are drawn.

Some students are fully supported by their organisations; they have leadership buy-in and ownership of AT as a core part of the organisations' offering. This leads to improved AT training and development and active engagement in improving the wider AT service. However, it is not always straightforward, as there is large variance in the AT maturity of organisations and very different expectations are made of the AT role. There can be differences in terms of budget support, ability to buy assessment equipment and limited budget for additional staff as the AT service scales. The EduAT team have seen occasional concerns with other professionals or groups around accepting the need for a 'professionalised AT role' in the unfounded belief that this may encroach on existing roles.

More experienced colleagues are, in part, studying the MSc EduAT because they want to improve recognition for a professional AT role within their own organisation. For those starting out with AT, the course can provide knowledge skills and understanding to undertake assessment, provisioning and ongoing support of AT in a range of organisations. There is now a 'formal' route into AT training for those who wish to train as an Assistive Technologist; this means students can develop as an Assistive Technologist or embed AT skills into another role such as teacher, technologist or allied health professional (primarily speech and language therapy or occupational therapy). In some organisations our student may be the only person who is working to support AT, in others they may be part of a wider AT team. The EduAT team have experience of a wide range of examples of how AT is implemented in the UK. There is also variation in where AT is located in organisational structures, sometimes within education teams, therapy services, IT or within a dedicated AT or a broader technology team. In some organisations we see good management buy in, and in others this is very difficult. The EduAT team have supported students and their management teams to embed the Assistive Technologist role and have signposted other services such as TechAbility and Jisc.[10,11] This support has been informal in some cases, and organisations have also engaged members of the programme team in a consultancy capacity to provide more time-intensive or targeted support for AT improvement programmes. The programme team have also formally supported the recruitment of AT roles. This has included support for the development of role and person specifications, development of candidate assessments, panel interviews and ongoing post-employment support and mentoring.

A useful feature of the course is the peer review and development that has taken place through an active learning set within the student body. Students have collaborated offline and have in some cases supported each other through peer review and development visits to each other's organisations and to provide assistance with difficult assessment cases, or to provide support with specific technical developments. The programme team plans to support the alumni of the course by converting existing digital spaces into an alumni resource that former students can access following graduation to network with peers and to access updated MSc EduAT teaching resources as the programme team continues to develop the programme.

An idea whose time has come?

In considering why it is a good time to professionalise the AT role now, this is partly due to the improvements in the underlying technology, in terms of reliability, cost and acceptance, factors that provide opportunities to an increasing number of people who might benefit. These opportunities can only be taken full advantage of if those using AT are supported to learn how to use it, alongside any supporting persons being trained to develop their understanding and ability to support the user and their technology.

Technology has improved with additional operating systems and productivity tools now having improved accessibility affordances and support for various access technologies such as switch access and eye-gaze natively 'baked into' the software. The expectations of users of AT have also been raised, in part due to the mainstreaming of accessible, lower-cost equipment. We should be clear that this mainstreaming of AT is not just about tablets and computers, it includes voice assistants, IoT (Internet of Things) technology and home automation or smart home-type technology used in place of higher-cost age and disability-badged ECS (environmental control systems). We can also include the mainstreaming of AI (artificial intelligence)-backed personal assistants and the potential of generative AI tools such as ChatGPT, Bard and Bing.

A Solution to a Difficult Problem?

The programme team, like many others, have been seeking a solution to the problem of having AT equipment and software in existence that is not being used to its potential for some time. This concern applies to both specialist and mainstream AT tools. The in-built accessibility options and affordances within mainstream operating systems and productivity tools continue to be iterated by the mainstream technology companies but few educators and other supporting staff understand how to use them. Specialist AT software and hardware have also been improved. The tools are better than ever; however, the specialists that are required to manage the assessment, provisioning and ongoing support of AT are not yet widely deployed. The problem of high-quality AT hardware and software existing, and supporting staff not knowing how to assess for, provision or deploy them and to provide the ongoing support for their use can be met by the AT role. Waller (2019) considered that:

> [The proposed role of the Assistive Technologist] is a new concept and a new professional cadre is required to realize it. There is a need for the training of Assistive Technologists which goes beyond the DART curriculum to include AAC training. Indeed, many online training and development resources already exist, e.g., the modules commissioned by the Scottish government based on the IPAACKS (Informing and Profiling AAC Knowledge and Skills) framework. However, there is a need to provide accredited training for a new profession who will work alongside other professionals to support and adapt the use of AT to meet the day-to-day needs of individuals, and those around them, in education, employment and in social settings. (p. 162)

Waller (2019) concluded that in relation to the provision of AAC technology the AT profession has a crucial role to play:

> Even when technology is innovated in collaboration with a wide range of stake-holders and identified by multidisciplinary teams, the adoption of AAC technology depends on a knowledgeable support environment. AAC technology is not an appliance which is plugged in and switched on. Instead it is a tool requiring ongoing support, ideally from Assistive Technologists working with educators and care staff to ensure that the true potential of AAC technology is realized! (p. 166)

The AT role is intended to pick up where a more generalised level of AT support provided by other professionals is no longer sufficient. Advocating for universal usability or universal adoption of accessible learning materials is an important factor, but it is not where efforts should stop. The concept of ordinary-extraordinary user design (Newell & Cairns, 1993) asserts that by meeting the requirements of users with the most complex needs, interfaces will be easier to use by everyone. This premise has underpinned the research and teaching within Computing at the University of Dundee for over three decades and has motivated an inclusive approach to the design of digital AT. There are, however, limits to what can be achieved with universal service delivery. You may be able to meet the needs of most, and not all users by advocating for a universal design approach; however, being inclusive does not mean treating everyone in the same way.

The UDL (Universal Design for Learning) approach has much to commend it (CAST, 2018); however, there are some limits to this approach. It may not be possible to meet the needs of all students via a UDL-type approach, even though you may meet the needs of many. Perhaps the most useful part of the UDL framework are the points related to the design of 'accessible educational materials'. The concept of ensuring that all educational materials are born accessible holds great value. It is crucial that educational materials are accessible so that an AT user may access them; for example, a screen reader user cannot access an inaccessible PDF document that is formulated using scanned images of text.

The UDL approach is viewed as complex, it is open to challenge and hard to measure the impact of a given element as Boysen (2021) so clearly articulates:

> If the premise of UDL sounds familiar, it is because it also happens to be the central idea of learning styles […]. In fact, UDL shares a startling number of similarities with the now discredited concept of learning styles. These similarities do not necessarily mean that the approach is ineffective or that it should be abandoned, especially as an accommodation for disability. However, critical analysis of overlap between the approaches is essential so that educators, theorists, and researchers do not make the same mistakes with UDL as they did with learning styles. (p. 2)

Boysen also quotes earlier work from Edyburn (2010), who commented on the difficulties on measuring the outcomes of UDL:

> Having multiple measures of learning within a single intervention makes it difficult to determine if UDL is effective (Edyburn, 2010). In addition, UDL presents students with multiple modes of representation and engagement. Thus, demonstrations of effectiveness need to account for the fact that implementations will inherently contain "multiple concurrent interventions" and multiple outcomes (Edyburn, 2010, p. 39). Overall, the complexity of UDL leaves a Gordian knot that researchers have not yet untangled in studies of the framework's effectiveness. (p. 7)

Universal Design For Learning may be helpful as an approach, especially with respect to the provision of accessible educational materials for students with specific requirements; however, as the approach cannot meet the needs of people with more complex needs there is a risk that some leaders may think that the approach solves all accessibility and AT provision requirements. An additional service level, beyond that offered by universal approaches such as UDL, is required for people with more complex needs. This is where the AT role is critical. Reducing AT abandonment is also an important factor which the person-centred approach at the core of the EduAT approach supports through asking the individual AT user what they wish to achieve and addressing those factors first. The problem we are seeking to address with the AT role is how to ensure the provision of high-quality user-centred AT services. An Assistive Technologist can assess for, provide and support the use of additional accommodations and technologies to enable a user to access materials that have been provided in an accessible format. This approach is closely allied to the ideas set out by Jewell and Atkin (2013: p. 17) in their report *Enabling Technologies*. Their recommendation to "allow the experience to be customised" can also be reframed as providing the hooks or digital affordances in product or system design. This can include accessible educational materials. Given accessible materials, then the Assistive Technologist may function as the 'chief integrator' of the technology system used by the user to access whatever they require. The UDL-type approach may not be effective for 'edge cases', or to put it another way, for people who have additional specific needs. This may mean that we can ask the question: is it even still a universal approach?

This open approach to extensible technology is helpful to those in the AT role as they can utilise the digital hooks or affordances to enable access through whatever input methods or tools may be appropriate and may even build new experiences upon the affordances provided. The recent experience in the education sector of having to move to online delivery during the Covid-19 pandemic has stimulated interest in accessibility from across the sector. Indeed, post-pandemic we have seen an increase in the demand and the need for digital skills, digital inclusion in general and the required accessibility improvements across digital platforms.

Funding the Future

There are not enough people working to support AT in education and beyond, as can be evidenced by the difficulties many organisations face when recruiting Assistive Technologists. There is a need to support training for people who wish to become Assistive Technologists. As a programme team we have supported the development of an EduAT scholarship that has been both charitably and corporately funded. This scholarship has been heavily oversubscribed, with applicants noting that without this support they cannot be supported by their organisations to access the course, due to increasing budgetary pressures. The MSc EduAT scholarship is a competitive process, with submissions assessed against an application essay rubric by a sub-group of the independent EduAT advisory group. It can also be identified that of the unsuccessful applicants, most do not otherwise find a way to access the course. This is a concern, as smaller organisations may not be able to access this professional development route due to budget concerns.

Once people are trained, it is useful for them to have a funded role to go to. We are aware that many organisations are not able to prioritise the budget to provide dedicated AT roles, even where the evidence of efficacy and therefore benefit to users of AT is accepted, primarily due to increasing pressure on budgets. We propose that by combining both support for training and support for AT roles in suitable organisations this downward spiral could be broken, with a trained workforce able to provide support to colleagues and AT users alike.

The Wider AT Support Context

Interestingly the calls for additional Assistive Technologists came at the same time as a reduction in the levels of sector-wide support available nationally in the UK from sector membership bodies and other organisations who previously provided AT support.

We would argue that there is a need for a new pan-sector AT-focused support body to replace the education sector support bodies that have been lost. A number of organisations have historically supported AT in education, such as the Special Education Microelectronic Resource Centres (Seale, 2022), Jisc TechDis (ETF, 2023) and the Jisc RSCs (Regional Support Centres), which provided AT, accessibility and inclusion support to higher and further education organisations and to the skills sector (Soares, 2014); the Brite Initiative, which provided AT support for Further Education Colleges in Scotland (Brite Initiative, 2014); and the British Educational Technology Agency (Becta), which provided AT support to schools and others (Becta, 2011). All of these organisations provided both formal and informal staff development opportunities for people who were working to support the use of AT in their organisations. This reduction in support again provided a driver for the development of a course to prepare people to be educational Assistive Technologists, as so many formal and informal development opportunities for those supporting AT are no longer available thanks to the losses of the support bodies noted earlier. All of these organisations no longer exist, due to the 'project' or short-term nature of the service funding, and the resulting 'gap' in support is clear to those who have worked in the AT and education sectors for some time. Indeed, in the early part of the first author's career the support provided by these organisations had a significant impact on individual and organisational

AT practice development. It can be argued that as a result of these losses the AT sector has seen a 'generational gap' where younger practitioners have not been identified, supported and developed in their AT-related careers. Indeed the losses in AT support also extend to the reduction in specialist advisory teachers in some local authorities.

The National Centre for AT that was proposed as part of the now defunct National Strategy for Disabled People (Disability Unit, 2022a; McLaren, 2021), or something like it, may be included in a future iteration of the Disability Action Plan (Disability Unit, 2022b), which has effectively replaced the National Strategy for Disabled People. It is possible that should the National Centre for AT, or an equivalent entity, become a service delivery organisation, this could provide the context for a national, UK-wide, pan-sector AT support body.

Today there are very few places for people who support AT in education and beyond to go for AT support, other than potentially the AT suppliers. This is not optimal as many suppliers do not have a sufficient account management or training function to practically support a large number of enquiries, and also some may have an assumed or actual proclivity to promote their products over products that may be more suitable for a given individual or group of users.

The first author has advocated for the support of the Natspec TechAbility service, which is part funded by the Karten Trust.[12,13] In part, the creation of the Natspec TechAbility service was advocated for due to the losses outlined earlier. Without a national support body for AT it is much more difficult for AT efforts to be nationally coordinated and supported. It is also difficult for policy makers to understand the 'situation on the ground' and to make good (evidence-based) decisions about future AT-related policy. It is suggested that the proposed AT support body could have service delivery, advice and guidance and national coordinating functions. This would enable those who are actively supporting AT users and colleagues across the various parts of the UK to provide useful feedback to ensure that policy makers and decision makers within the civil service at all levels could obtain useful intelligence with which to aid future decision-making and service delivery.

Potential Solutions to the Problems of both Professionalising AT and Coordinating Support for AT Efforts

We believe that in order for AT to reach its potential in the UK a number of things must happen simultaneously:

1. Ringfenced funding support is required for training, at all levels and not just for professional-level courses such as MSc EduAT. Support must include entry-level and intermediate continuing professional development (CPD) courses.

2. Once people are trained, they must have AT roles to move into. It is important therefore to support ringfenced funding for AT specialist posts in a variety of contexts. This can include specialist colleges and special schools, general further education colleges and universities, as well as various social care and third sector contexts. Such contexts have the funding models and localised demand for AT to create specialist roles. In mainstream primary and secondary schools, and other smaller contexts, access to a AT specialist must, for reasons of economics or scale, be shared over multiple sites. In the education sector, this could perhaps be done within a multi-academy trust or within a local education authority. In other sectors other regionally defined structures would be required.

3. Thirdly, a national pan-sector (education, social care, health and other contexts) AT support organisation is required to support both specialists and people in other roles in a coherent way. Currently there are very few organisations for those working to support AT users to go for professional support themselves. Such a body has not existed cross-sector previously.

Without the aforementioned three actions taking place simultaneously or near to simultaneously it is suggested that it will be difficult to reverse the decline of available AT-related support nationally in the UK that has taken place over the last decade and previously.

A research agenda for AT

The Dundee AT/AAC Research Group has a long history of innovative AAC, AT and user-centred computing research (see Waller, 2019). The group plans to develop new projects as well as renewing some of the group's previous technology projects by developing research into replicable and scalable 'products' that the community may benefit from. Some of those new projects will be drawn from our experience of developing the MSc EduAT. The collective experience of the programme team has brought us to the conclusion that supporting the professionalisation of the Assistive Technologist role would be useful. We developed the MSc EduAT in order to provide such a profession-alisation route. The direct experience of developing and delivering the MSc EduAT and critically the experience gained through supporting our students have also led us to propose the development of three new research projects that are designed to address the challenges that have been further elucidated by this professionalisation effort. Perhaps most importantly each proposal is directly informed by the professionalisation effort. To put it another way, the proposals are designed to address problems that the programme team and our students are experiencing in the development and delivery of AT services in the UK context.

Proposal 1: Identifying the Social Return on Investment (SROI) Generated by Specialist AT Roles

This proposal is perhaps the most important, as it is focused on evidencing the impact of dedicated AT roles by investigating the social return on investment gained by society, AT-providing or -supporting organisations and critically the people who these organisations support to use AT. This project can be summarised as an interdisciplinary social return on investment project, aiming to inform evidence-based policy making.

It is acknowledged that in the UK context any incoming government drawn from any political parties will be facing difficult decisions on what to support with a limited resource. Any calls to support dedicated funding for AT posts and training will need to be backed up with evidence of efficacy to be taken seriously. There may also be opportunities to support the development of a service delivery organisation, to both learn from previous efforts and build upon them.

This project has been designed to address the need to evidence the impact of specialist AT roles such as the Assistive Technologist. In recent years there have been a number of AT-related policy developments that for various reasons have not come to fruition. The development of the proposed National Centre for AT, as discussed in the now defunct National Disability Strategy, has apparently stalled. This development has not yet been included in the replacement National Disability Action Plan. However, there remains a focus from government in the National Disability Action Plan on joining up efforts across departments to support disabled people.

This proposed project would support the increased prioritisation for AT development that has been in evidence in various government departments and organisations that support disabled people. Examples of improved join-up include the Department for Education's AT training pilots (Department for Education, 2022), which aimed to develop the AT skills of teachers and other staff in mainstream schools, and the Department for Work and Pensions Access to Work Passports (Department for Work and Pensions, 2021), which aimed to bridge the transition from university- and college-focused Disabled Student Allowance and employment.

The proposed research would focus on what the SROI (social return on investment) is, when specialist AT roles are introduced to an organisation such as a school, college, university or other research context. This project can consider quantitative data such as destinations, achievement rates and where possible exam or course pass rates. In addition there is value in specific stories or case studies as they can bring a richness to the lived experience of individuals, and it is acknowledged that it will be important not to represent these stories as data. This project will aim to understand the difference that the Assistive Technologist role makes to organisations, teams and individuals, in terms of changed student outcomes, destination data, etc. It may be useful to undertake a medium-to-long term project looking at the impact of the AT role on organisations in order to ensure that changes are sustained, and subsequent policy proposals can be evidenced appropriately.

It is thought to be helpful to clearly evidence the impact of AT roles, as it will be difficult to validate further investment in training and ringfenced funding for organisations to resource AT posts and for support around the creation of a national AT support organisation. The latter could underpin all related activity and link what is happening 'on the ground' to enable decision makers to be clearly informed. Note the clear links here to two of the recommendations made by Edyburn (2020) regarding AT training for specialists and connecting AT input to AT outcomes.

This work will be interdisciplinary; therefore, beyond computing/AT researchers, this project can involve colleagues within:

1. *Education:* Many of those in an AT role work in education contexts. We plan to consider if changes/improvements to educational outcomes as a result of high-quality AT assessment, provisioning and ongoing support might lead to improved achievement rates and destinations, inclusive of further study, and ultimately employment and resulting economic activity.

This would be a medium-to-long term (possibly longitudinal) study and can also consider historical data where these exist.

2. *Health and social care:* A health economist could help calculate potential savings. For example, when a person with physical disabilities is taught or trained to use environmental controls and other AT, how does this potentially impact on their lifetime cost of care? This must be approached with caution, to avoid ethical concerns such as social isolation or other risks of harm, should human support be inappropriately replaced with technology.

3. *Humanities/social science:* Informed access to research methods from anthropology such as ethnographic surveys, can provide the richer human case studies/stories of how high-quality AT assessment, provisioning and ongoing support have had an impact on an individual or group.

The proposed project is informed by work to professionalise the Assistive Technologist role as we know that organisations find it difficult to fund both Assistive Technologist roles and the training such post holders require. Through undertaking this project it will be possible to elucidate the impact such roles have in order to support the case for ringfenced funding for AT posts, AT training and ultimately a pan-sectoral support body that can underpin all AT work nationally.

Proposal 2: AT Assessment Tool Development

We propose the building of a web-based AT assessment (ATA) software tool to support suitably qualified and experienced staff to undertake high-quality needs-based assessment. It is not intended to replace people with AT skills, rather to support them. Based on feedback from MSc EduAT students, undertaking AT assessment is an area that they need support to develop. By having a branching logic underpinning the assessment tool it will be possible to support the assessment process through the inclusion of prompt questions that will support decision-making. The documentation of assessment and the creation of support documentation could be partially automated, as this is another area that EduAT students have identified as difficult, with some describing that they do not have formalised AT assessment policies, procedures or documentation in place. Such an effort would reduce the need for each organisation to 'reinvent the wheel', in order to put a formal assessment process in place. The tool could scale with the complexity of the assessment and could point to statutory assessment routes where relevant. In this way developing professionals could be supported to access expert support.

The aim is for the same tool to be useful for assessments undertaken at multiple educational stages, levels, ages, and transition points, and for it to output useful reporting and guidance materials (e.g., AT or AAC passports), or training and support materials for staff members who will be setting up or preparing AT equipment or software for the AT user.

The aims of creating an ATA tool can include:

1. Reducing abandonment of AT.
2. Being genuinely person-centred, including prioritisation of what the user wants to do (first!).
3. Reducing administrative burden on Assistive Technologists and the organisations that they work within.

Being genuinely person-centred is extremely important with respect to reducing AT abandonment. Any tool must start from the user's requirement and work from there, in order for user acceptance to be paramount. The expectation is that this ATA tool will also include a knowledge base of available AT. This will be a significant undertaking to create in the first instance and would also need to be regularly updated to continue to be useful. Early answers or selections in the ATA tool will inform the path through a branching tree logic diagram, informing the proposed methods of a given AT assessment and the tools suggested for trial. It is a high priority for the tool to be used to bridge 'transition stages' (school to college, college to university, school or college to work, etc.). The reason for this is to reduce the time spent repeating previous steps, which will save both the AT user's time, and will give the AT assessor intelligence so that their new work may be informed by any previous work.

It would be helpful to include a 'log' for the staff team undertaking the ATA and should outputs also include training or set-up materials for those supporting the user, this will save significant time as such documentation would not need to constantly be re-created, thereby also reducing some of the opportunity for abandonment if the staff team around the user are able to support the technology in an informed way. As a consequence of creating a knowledge base of available AT systems there may also be some additional opportunities to standardise how accessibility information is presented for each tool. It is critical that the development of this tool be informed by disabled people's experiences. To this end it is proposed that all development be co-produced or better yet co-investigated by disabled people.

Proposal 3: Developing an AT Framework and Discovery Tool

The Educational Assistive Technologist is not the only post that supports the use of AT; indeed part of the vision for the EduAT role is to train the trainer. Many other members of staff in various organisations require a level of knowledge around AT, and they require training. Not every organisation that provides AT support needs or can afford to employ a specialist Assistive Technologist. The EduAT programme team do not believe that all those working to support AT require a Masters level qualification. The EduAT programme team, members of the advisory group and students have identified that it can be difficult to find the right course to meet a specific need.

Our third proposal focuses on improving the discoverability of AT resources and training through the design of an AT training framework that identifies what training is needed by people in a range of roles, in different organisational contexts and at different stages of their AT journey. We propose that this can be achieved by developing a web-based tool that catalogues all of the AT training and resources available within commercial, education, health and social care contexts. The web-based AT training and resource discovery tool would require some scaffolding to ensure that useful courses and resources were presented to people who are working in various roles in different types of organisations and at various stages of their AT learning journey. To that end the development of an AT framework is proposed. It could be based on the existing AAC specific IPAACKS (NHS Education for Scotland, 2014) tool, but would need to be broader in terms of the types of AT covered and the levels of awareness or competences. This would require the inclusion of an additional level 0 'awareness raising' level (i.e., below level 1 in the current framework). The available AT training and resources would be stored in a database and can be mapped onto this framework, using simple metadata to identify for whom they may be useful. The process by which existing courses are identified and catalogued with metadata to enable them to be selected by the web-based tool's system logic would also enable training gaps to be identified, enabling future AT training course development to be targeted in an informed way.

The proposed web-based tool would ask simple questions, including: where do you work, what is your role and what is your AT awareness/learning level? The output from this would be a proposed pathway, with links to the various training options and resources offered by various organisations. In this way the web tool could be used by colleagues from a variety of organisations to support the discoverability of AT resources and training at multiple levels. This project would output the AT training framework, the web-based AT training and resource discovery tool and an analysis of where the gaps in training provision might be.

Conclusions

This chapter has aimed to consider how the experience of the EduAT programme team, our advisory group and the input of our three cohorts of
students gained through the development and delivery of the MSc EduAT
has informed our AT research agenda. We have described how and why we
built the MSc EduAT. We have reflected on what we have learned from our
students as we have developed and delivered the sole AT-focused MSc in the
UK. Finally we have gone on to discuss what research may be required in order
to support future development of high-quality AT service delivery.

It is concluded that support for training alone is not enough; this must be
supported by funding for posts in organisations that assess for, provide and
support AT. The Assistive Technologist post holders and many other professionals who also support AT users can be effectively aided by a national,
pan-sector AT support body. Should these elements be enacted together it is
possible for the entire enterprise to be more effective.

In order to make the case for these interventions at a policy level, it is essential
that the underpinning AT research is developed. By evidencing the impact of
the Assistive Technologist role and other similar AT specialist roles through
the proposed social return on investment project we can help build the evidence base. This work supports policy development that can improve funding
for specialist AT posts and the training that such posts require. This work
can provide the due diligence or assurances to decision makers that such an
investment will have a useful impact on the quality of life, and positive life
outcomes for all of the disabled people who might benefit from AT. It will not
be possible to provide such evidence without conducting research to demonstrate the impact of the AT role, to show the social return on investment. By
developing transdisciplinary research methods, quality assurance and service
improvement methods and metrics, the impact of the transdisciplinary AT
role can be quantified. We propose that by equipping Assistive Technologists
with an AT assessment tool they will be supported to undertake high-quality
person-centred AT assessments. Assessments that are focused on what the AT
user wishes to achieve may support a reduction in AT abandonment, hence
the proposal to develop a supportive AT assessment tool. In order to develop
the AT skills, knowledge and practice a range of professionals, in a variety of
organisations, who are at different stages of their AT journey we propose the
development of an AT training framework onto which available AT training
opportunities can be mapped. Having done this, it will be useful to create
a web-based tool to render such training discoverable and to present it in a way

that is highly relevant to the user of the tool. Additionally the act of creating the framework and the discovery tool will illuminate gaps in provision.

Our proposals to undertake this work are born out of our professional experience and our recent focus on the development and delivery of the MSc EduAT. This work has been closely informed by the experience of AT users, our students and colleagues. We would like to work together collegiately with colleagues from the UK and beyond to realise this proposed work for the advantage of everyone who can benefit from AT. We encourage users of AT, disabled people, academic colleagues, postgraduate students and researchers, professionals working in education, health, social care and beyond to support this effort. The EduAT programme team welcomes contact from any interested persons to constructively comment on, improve or extend our proposals. By conducting practically focused, outcome-driven, co-designed, or better yet, co-investigated research that is driven by AT users and disabled peoples' experiences, we can ensure that the potential of AT is realised for everyone who can benefit.

Notes

1 Rehabilitation Engineering and AT Society of North America: Get Certified: https://www.resna.org/Certification
2 Dundee University User Centre: https://aac.dundee.ac.uk/user-centre/
3 All-Party Parliamentary Group for AT, Policy Connect: https://www.policyconnect.org.uk/appgat
4 Rehabilitation Engineering and Assistive Technologies MSc: https://www.ucl.ac.uk/prospective-students/graduate/taught-degrees/rehabilitation-engineering-and-assistive-technologies-msc
5 Natspec is a UK membership association for organisations that offer specialist further education and training for students with learning difficulties and/or disabilities aged 16 to 25: https://natspec.org.uk/
6 Beaumont College: https://www.beaumontcollege.ac.uk/
7 College Development Network: https://www.cdn.ac.uk/
8 Care Quality Commission: https://www.cqc.org.uk/
9 Ofsted: https://www.gov.uk/government/organisations/ofsted
10 TechAbility: https://www.techability.org.uk/
11 Jisc: https://www.jisc.ac.uk/
12 Karten Trust: https://iankartencharitabletrust.org.uk/
13 Note that the author is a trustee of the Karten Network, which is related to the Karten charity, and therefore declares an interest.

References

Becta (2011). *Announcement on the future of Becta.* https://webarchive.nationalarchives .gov.uk/ukgwa/20110125133530mp_/http://news.becta.org.uk/display.cfm?resID= 42305

Boysen, G. (2021). Lessons (not) learned: The troubling similarities between learning styles and universal design for learning. *Scholarship of Teaching and Learning in Psychology.* https://doi.org/10.1037/stl0000280.

Brite Initiative (2014). *The BRITE blog.* https://briteblog.wordpress.com/

CAST (2018). *Universal Design for Learning Guidelines version 2.2.* https://udlguidelines .cast.org/

Department for Education (2022). *AT training pilot evaluation.* Retrieved 6 July 2023 from: https://www.gov.uk/government/publications/assistive-technology-training -pilot-evaluation

Department for Work and Pensions (2021). *New government 'passport' to help disabled graduates get in to employment.* Retrieved 6 July 2023 from: https://www.gov.uk/ government/news/new-government-passport-to-help-disabled-graduates-get-in-to -employment

Disability Unit (2022a). *National Disability Strategy.* Retrieved 4 July 2023 from: https://www.gov.uk/government/publications/national-disability-strategy

Disability Unit (2022b). *New Disability Action Plan confirmed for 2023 as minister meets Paralympians and opens pioneering lab at Olympic Park.* Retrieved 4 July 2023 from: https://www.gov.uk/government/news/new-disability-action-plan-confirmed -for-2023-as-minister-meets-paralympians-and-opens-pioneering-lab-at-olympic -park

Edyburn, D. (2020). *Rapid literature review on AT in education.* https://assets.publishing .service.gov.uk/government/uploads/system/uploads/attachment_data/file/937381/ UKAT_FinalReport_082520.pdf

Edyburn, D.L. (2010). Would you recognize universal design for learning if you saw it? Ten propositions for new directions for the second decade of UDL. *Learning Disability Quarterly, 33*(1), 33–41. https://doi.org/10.1177/073194871003300103

ESCO (2022). *Assistive Technologist.* https:// esco .ec .europa .eu/ en/ classification/ occupation ?uri = http:// data .europa .eu/ esco/ occupation/ 4e82464b -e9d7–4d51–9116–294ab40c5169

ETF (2023). *About the JISC TechDis approach.* https://toolkits.excellencegateway.org .uk/about-jisc-techdis-approach

Jewell, S., & Atkin, R. (2013). *Enabling Technology.* Royal College of Art: The Helen Hamlyn Centre for Design. http://rossatkin.com/docs/Enabling_Technology_lo_res %20FINAL.pdf

Maudslay, L. (2015). *AT in further education organisations 2014–15.* https://repository .jisc.ac.uk/6243/1/NATSPEC-report-Oct15.pdf

McLaren, R. (2021). *The National Disability Strategy: Tech is the opportunity, collaboration its realisation. Policy Connect.* Retrieved 4 July 2023 from: https:// www .policyconnect .org .uk/ blog/ national -disability -strategy -tech -opportunity -collaboration-its-realisation

Natspec (2023). *TechAbility Standards.* https:// www .techability .org .uk/ techability -standards/

Newell, A.F., & Cairns, A.Y. (1993). Designing for extraordinary users. *Ergonomics in Design, 1*(4), 10–16. https://doi.org/10.1177/106480469300100405

NHS Education for Scotland (2014). *IPAACKS: Informing and profiling AAC knowledge and skills*. MHS Education for Scotland. https://www.aacscotland.org.uk/files/cm/files/ipaacks.pdf

Ofsted (2015). *Developing active communication skills: Royal College Manchester*. Retrieved 3 July 2023 from: https:// www .gov .uk/ government/ publications/ developing-active-communication-skills-royal-college-manchester

Seale, J. (2022). *Technology Use by Adults with Learning Disabilities: Past, Present and Future Design and Support Practice*. Routledge.

Seale, J., & Turner-Smith, A. (2001). Multidisciplinary Postgraduate Education in AT: Challenges and Opportunities. *Proceedings of the RESNA 2001 Annual Conference* (pp. 196–198). RESNA Press.

Slaughter, R., & Mobbs, T. (2015). The DART Project: Improving AT provision in further education. *Communication Matters Journal, 29*(2), 24–26.

Soares, G. (2014). *News: RSCl8trs marks the end of RSC London at ULCC. JISC RSC London*. https://jiscrsclondon.wordpress.com/category/news/

University of Dundee (2023). *Teaching and assessment – Educational AT (part-time) MSc*, University of Dundee. https:// www .dundee .ac .uk/ postgraduate/ educational -assistive-technology-part-time/teaching-and-assessment

Waller, A. (2019). Telling tales: Unlocking the potential of AAC technologies. *International Journal of Language & Communication Disorders, 54*(2), 159–169. https://doi.org/10.1111/1460-6984.12449

Whitney, G., Suzette, K., Buhler, C., Hewer, S., Lhotska, L., Miesenberger, K., Sandnes, F.E., Stephanidis, C., & Velasco, C.A. (2011). Twenty five years of training and education in ICT Design for All and AT. *Technology and Disability, 23*(3), 163–170. https://doi.org/10.3233/TAD-2011-0324

WHO (2023). *AT*. Retrieved 4 July 2023 from: https://www.who.int/news-room/fact -sheets/detail/assistive-technology

9. Methods for achieving greater involvement of people with disabilities in the design of technologies

Jane Seale

Introduction: how should we respond to the call for more involvement of people with disabilities?

In Chapter 1 I noted that there was a call from both policy actors and research-ers for more user involvement in the design of assistive technologies (ATs). Those making such calls wrote as if the disability and technology community had a shared understanding of what greater 'user involvement' means and how to achieve this. I have learnt from experience that this is not necessarily the case. Between 2016 and 2019 I was involved in a three-year European project called ARCHES that aimed to create more inclusive cultural environments for adults who have a range of access preferences through the development of new technologies. The project partners included technology companies, museums and researchers. The project was positioned as participatory in that people with sensory and intellectual disabilities were involved in evaluating their museum experiences and in designing the new technologies. At the end of the first year we realised that everyone's understanding of participation was different and this was causing tensions. The technology partners were used to focusing their products and research upon specific impairment categories and to having a more quantitative, quasi-experimental expectation of participation. This was contrary to the way the researchers and the participants wanted to work, which initially caused some tensions (see Travnicek et al., 2022). The aim of this chapter is to examine the extent to which a shared understanding of user involvement exists across the wider disability and technology community. In particular it will seek answers to the following questions:

1. What approaches are commonly used to involve people with disabilities in the design of new technologies?

2. What factors influence the decisions regarding which design approach to adopt?
3. Is there any evidence that one particular approach to involving users in design is more effective than another or produces more effective (e.g., accessible, acceptable, usable) AT?
4. How can AT developers be supported to enhance the involvement of users with disabilities?

I will begin by providing an overview of the approaches that are most commonly used to include users in the design of technologies. I will then review design studies conducted between 2018 and 2023 that have attempted to apply these common design approaches to the design of technologies for people with disabilities. In particular, I will critique the factors that have influenced the choice of these two approaches and identify challenges and issues that can inform a future research agenda in the field of disability and technology.

What approaches are used to include users in the design of technologies?

A logical first step is to look at common approaches to including users in the design of technologies and ascertain whether they have been or have the potential to be applied to the design of technologies for people with disabilities. For the purposes of this chapter I am defining a design approach as an overarching philosophy or set of principles for involving users that is intended to guide designers towards a particular end-goal. Approaches for involving users in the design of technologies are not prescriptive and do not specify exact tools or techniques that should be used to achieve the end-goal, although some particular tools and techniques tend to be more commonly associated with particular design approaches than others.

There are a number of approaches to including users in the process of researching and designing of technologies, but the two most commonly employed ones appear to be User-centred Design and Participatory Design (see for example a review by Seale et al., 2020). User-centred Design (UCD) and Participatory Design (PD) are distinguishable from Universal Design, Barrier-free Design, Design for All, Accessible Design and Inclusive Design, because they focus on the process of designing rather than the end product of the design process. Designers who use UCD and PD might opt to use approaches such as Universal Design at some point in the design journey, but they do not form a core part of the UCD or PD overarching design philosophy. It is also important to distinguish UCD from UXD (User Experience Design). UXD is the process of designing products that are useful, easy to use and a pleasure to engage with. It is about enhancing the entire experience people have while interacting with a product, and making sure they find value and satisfaction in the product. A good user experience (UX) is an intended outcome of UCD. However, UX is just one aspect that UCD focuses on. Designers who use the UCD approach may therefore incorporate UXD frameworks or methods (e.g., Design Thinking or Double Diamond) as part of a wider repertoire of frameworks, tools and techniques.

The key differences and similarities between UCD and PD are summarised in Table 9.1. In the following sections I will provide a more detailed overview of the two approaches to involving users in the design of technologies.

Table 9.1   Similarities and differences between User-centred Design and Participatory Design

Issues considered		UCD	PD
What	Underpinning principles	Improving the understanding of user and task requirements	Democracy Interactive two-way relationship between designer and user
	Key focus or overarching characteristics	Usability	Collaboration
Why	Main goals and/or motivations	A better product A better user experience	A better product A better quality of life (through use of end product)
Who	Who are the actors in the design process?	End-users and designers/developers	Designers/developers, end-users, relevant external stakeholders
	How are the end-users of the product or service being designed/ conceptualised?	Informants (providing feedback) Subject	Partners Active/full participant Co-designer Decision maker
How	Processes	Iterative	Iterative
	Commonly used tools and techniques	Task analysis, needs analysis, usability testing, think aloud protocols, heuristic evaluation, prototyping (lo-tech, rapid)	Collages, mappings and mock-ups; diaries and card sorting tasks; games, acting, or improvisation

User-centred Design

It is generally accepted that the focus of UCD is on usability (Preece et al., 1994) in order to get a better understanding of users and task requirements (Nelson et al., 2013; Mao et al., 2005). UCD typically involves the user in the development cycle, obtaining their feedback on early designs and redesigning prototypes in light of user feedback and comments. Many user-centred designers point to the usability principles proposed by Gould and Lewis (1985) which emphasise early focus on users and tasks, empirical measurement and iterative design. With regards to early focus, UCD designers must understand who the users will be. This understanding is arrived at in part by directly studying their cognitive, behavioural, anthropometric and attitudinal characteristics, and in part by studying the nature of the work expected to be accomplished. In terms of empirical measurement, intended users in a UCD project are required to actually use simulations and prototypes to carry out real work, and their performance and reactions are observed, recorded and analysed. Finally, when problems are found in user testing, they must be fixed through a cycle of design, test and measure, and redesign. This is repeated as often as necessary.

A range of tools and techniques are used within the UCD approach. For example, Abras et al. (2004) give examples such as task and needs analysis, prototyping, background interviews and questionnaires, focus groups, on-site observation, role-playing walkthroughs, simulations and usability testing. Mao et al. (2005) list user requirement analysis, task analysis, focus groups, formal heuristic evaluation, user interviews, surveys and card sorting. Nelson et al. (2013) suggests that a usability assessment will involve usability testing, inspection methods, expert surveys, interviews and focus groups and that none of these methods on their own will produce sufficient information on usability.

Participatory Design

Generally speaking, PD (sometimes referred to as co-design or cooperative design) is understood as the collaboration of designers and non-designers in the design of products and services (Sanders & Stappers, 2008; Greenbaum & Kyng, 1991). Non-designers are potential users as well as other relevant stakeholders such as carers, service providers, engineers or marketing and sales professionals (Sanders et al., 2010). In positioning non-professional designers (users) as collaborators, PD researchers frequently refer to them as co-designers, partners and full or active participants (Muller & Druin, 2012). The need for active participation is also emphasised; something more than being used as mere data sources by responding to questionnaires or being observed while using the software (Muller & Kuhn, 1993). As partners or co-designers, users offer their expertise regarding their needs, experiences and evaluations of products. Their knowledge and skills are recognised alongside the knowledge and skills of the professional designers (Blomberg & Henderson, 1990). The goal or intended outcome of PD is to improve the quality of life for users by providing them with better-quality products or services.

Participatory design started in the 1970s with a focus on worker participations in decisions about technologies. Over time it has evolved towards a broader focus on users rather than workers and encompassing a broader range of artefacts/products (Bødker et al., 1993). However, the commitment to user involvement in the decision-making remains. The willingness to accept users as experts and partners is underpinned by a commitment to democratic design and a rejection of 'patriarchy' (Ellis & Kurniawan, 2000). Users are afforded the right to be actively involved in decisions that will affect their quality of life/work. Integral to being a partner in the design process is being a decision maker (Carroll et al., 2000; Muller & Kuhn, 1993).

In order for users to meaningfully influence design decisions some PD researchers argue that ideally they need to be involved both early in and throughout the design process, including the initiation of the design idea (ideation) and analysis of the evaluation/usability data (Ellis & Kurniawan, 2000; Muller et al., 1997). Muller et al. (1997), however, argue that the reality is somewhat different and that the timing of when user influence happens is highly variable.

The process of sharing knowledge is seen as two-way (interactive exchange) where both designer and non-designer learn something new (Muller & Druin, 2012). Collaboration between designer and user is also positioned as iterative, where emerging designs are tried out with users, and their experiences (often in the real world) inform future versions of the design (Blomberg & Henderson, 1990). PD also values interactive evaluation to gather and integrate feedback from intended users, thereby promoting design iteration (Ellis & Kurniawan, 2000).

A range of tools and techniques are used within the PD approach such as scenarios, mock-up simulations, future workshops and design games (Kensing & Blomberg, 1998; Bødker et al., 1993). Like UCD, PD uses prototyping but differentiates it from UCD by calling it cooperative or participatory prototyping. Like UCD, PD employs questionnaires, interviews and focus groups, but places less emphasis on using these techniques as part of a structured task or needs analysis. Sanders et al. (2010) delineate between PD methods that involve making tangible things (e.g., 2D collages or 3D mock-ups); methods that involve talking, telling or explaining (e.g., diaries or the use of cards to organise, categorise and prioritise ideas); and methods involving acting or playing (e.g., game-boards, improvisations and play acting). Muller et al. (1997) distinguish between PD methods that are employed within the user's world such as ethnography, Forum Theatre and mock-ups; methods that are employed within the designer's world such as prototyping and workshops; and methods that occupy the space in-between these two worlds such as scenarios and storytelling.

Distinguishing between the Common Approaches to Including Users in the Design of Technologies

The major difference between PD and UCD is the role that the user takes in the design process. Although there will be variations within each approach, generally speaking users in a PD project will be more involved in the design decisions and therefore will be more likely to be considered a member of the design team compared to UCD (Dirks, 2019). However, distinguishing between the two approaches is complicated by a number of factors. Firstly, there are a number of similarities between the two approaches: such as the involvement of the user throughout the design process and using iterative design processes. Secondly, definitions of approaches do not always explicitly highlight what makes one approach different from another. Thirdly, it is acknowledged that one approach can influence another, which can result in designers blurring the distinctions:

> The user-centered design approach (i.e., "user as subject") has been primarily a US driven phenomenon. Increasingly, since the 70s, people have been given more influence and room for initiative in roles where they provide expertise, and participate in the informing, ideating, and conceptualizing activities in the early design phases. The participatory approach (i.e. "user as partner") has been led by Northern Europeans. The two approaches are now beginning to influence one another. (Sanders & Stappers, 2008, p. 5)

One major consequence of the difficulties in distinguishing between the two approaches is that developers can (incorrectly in my view) position one approach as a sub-set or extension of the other. For example, Abras et al. (2004: p. 456) state: "A variety of methods have been developed to support UCD including usability testing, usability engineering, heuristic evaluation, discount evaluation and participatory design".

If designers are going to blur the distinctions between UCD and PD, it is my contention that they need to provide a justification for such blurring. Without such justification, it would seem reasonable to assume that designers do not have a full comprehension of the history behind each approach and there-fore the very different design aims and outcomes. Furthermore, if we allow the distinctions to become blurred, and for UCD and PD to be considered synonymous, then we risk losing the PD focus on users being involved in the design decision-making. Such agency and empowerment, I would argue, is an important indicator of digital inclusion (see Chapter 2 for a more extensive discussion of digital inclusion).

What approaches are used to include users with disabilities in the design of technologies?

UCD and PD were not developed with users with disabilities in mind, and some experts in the field consider this to be concerning with regards to ensuring the genuine participation of people with disabilities in the design of new technol-ogies. For example, Newell et al. (2011) argue that UCD methods provide little or no guidance about how to design for people with disabilities and that using traditional UCD is problematic when the user group includes some users with disabilities or is entirely composed of users with disabilities because it means there is a greater variety of user characteristics and functionality, which may mean it is difficult to find designs that suit users with and without disabilities or users with different kinds of access needs. Newell et al. (2011) suggest an extension to UCD that they call 'User-Sensitive Inclusive Design' which they argue requires designers to develop a real empathy for users with disabilities. They reject standard UCD methods such as usability tests and experiments where users are positioned as 'subjects' and instead highlight methods such as ethnography, personas, scenarios and theatrical techniques involving pro-fessional actors as useful and appropriate techniques to use with users with disabilities. However, there are very few examples in the literature of other designers adopting this proposed extension to UCD.

Given such tensions regarding the appropriateness of applying PD and UCD to the design of technologies for people with disabilities I would argue that it is important to interrogate in more detail how technology designers decide which design approach to use with users with disabilities; what, if any, justifi-cations they give for their choices; and what factors influence their choices. In this section I will report on an extensive but not exhaustive critical review of the literature that I undertook in order to identify challenges and issues that could inform a future research agenda in the field of disability and technology. In particular, I will use the critical review to address the following questions:

1. What factors influence the choice of approach to involve users with disabilities in the design of AT?
   a. What justifications are given for the choice of design approach?
   b. Are the approaches adapted in any particular way to make them more accessible to users with disabilities?
2. Is there any evidence that one particular design approach is more effective at involving users with disabilities or produces more effective (accessible, acceptable, usable) AT?
   a. What evaluative evidence is provided to demonstrate successful employment of a design approach with users with disabilities?
   b. What challenges are there in employing design approaches with users with disabilities?

I located the studies to be included in this critical review by searching the SCOPUS database for papers, book chapters and conference papers published between 2018 and 2023. The focus of the search was studies that described and/ or evaluated the process of designing a new technology for people with disabilities. Design-related literature reviews and discussion papers were excluded from the search. Studies were incorporated in the review if they referenced disability, technology and design/evaluation within the title, abstract or keywords. I also searched within the following journals that I knew included studies on disability and technology: *Disability and Society*; *JMIR Rehabilitation and Assistive Technologies*; *Assistive Technology*; *Journal of Enabling Technologies*; *Technology & Disability*; and *Disability and Rehabilitation: Assistive Technology*. Finally, to ensure appropriate coverage of computer science-related research I searched through assistive technology-related international conference proceedings published in the high-profile Lecture Notes in Computer Science series. I excluded several studies which had confusing or incorrect labelling of the design approach; for example, including both UCD and PD in the keywords but then not explicitly referring to either of these in the rest of the paper, or making a claim that PD is an example of UCD. Tables 9.2 to 9.4 provide an overview of the resulting studies. Where the studies indicated the size of the user group, this is indicated in parentheses.

Table 9.2   Overview of User-centred Design studies

Study	Discipline	Country	Technology	User group	Tools and techniques
Jie et al., 2020	Rehabilitation design and technology	Netherlands	Mobile app involving sensor feedback	Stroke and cognitive impairments (15)	Double diamond method Prototyping
Richardson et al., 2021	Rehabilitation science	Canada	Web-based tool	Patients with chronic conditions (11)	Usability test Heuristic evaluation Focus groups Think aloud method
Thirumalai et al., 2018	Health sciences Engineering	US	Video game for Wii Fit Balance Board	Wheelchair users – lower extremity mobility limitation	Iterative user testing
Grolier et al., 2023	Health/clinical sciences	France	Mobile app	Chronic low back pain (18)	User testing Questionnaires and interviews
	Health sciences Engineering	Netherlands	Telecare – wireless activity monitor	Elderly people (35)	Double diamond method Interviews Focus groups User testing in own home

Table 9.3   Overview of Participatory Design studies

Study	Discipline	Country	Technology	User group	Tools & techniques
Layton et al., 2021	Occupational therapy Physiotherapy Psychology	Australia	Service online peer community	AT users – varied (600)	Living Lab Approach Surveys Focus groups Journey mapping Think tanks
Ferati et al., 2018	Informatics	Sweden	Smart home/IoT	Mixed disabilities (6)	Cartographic mapping Future workshop Cultural probes
Joshi & Valen, 2018	Informatics	Norway	PC-related access technologies	Physical disability, rheumatoid disorders (64)	Group discussions Field notes Photographs Interviews Prototype testing
Allin et al., 2018	Health sciences	Canada	Internet-based self-management program	Spinal cord injury (9)	Consumer advisory group Prototyping
Garcia et al., 2021	Design informatics Computer science Engineering	Brazil	Sign language machine translation	Hearing impairments	Observation
Vollenwyder et al., 2020	Psychology	Switzerland	Mobile app	Visual impairments (36) Other users with disabilities (3)	Workshops Hackathon Prototype testing Questionnaire Usability testing

Study	Discipline	Country	Technology	User group	Tools & techniques
Williams & Gibson, 2020	Information studies	UK	Social media	Learning disabilities (53)	Surveys Focus groups
Kortekaas & Zorn, 2022	Applied sciences	Germany	Generic AT	Young people with additional needs, some with mild learning disabilities (6)	Workshop/conversation
Aswad et al., 2022	Computer science	Ireland	Accessible digital applications	Intellectual disabilities (15)	Focus groups
Waardenburg et al., 2021	Applied sciences Psychiatry Neuroscience	Netherlands	Unspecified technologies – no specific description	Young autistic adults (3)	Action-oriented tinkering User-initiated design Use of off-the shelf technologies
Cosentino et al., 2021	Science & technology	Norway/Italy	Smart outdoor experiences	Intellectual disabilities (4)	COBO toolkit Inspirational cards Interactive smart objects Multimedia
Harris et al., 2022	Computer science	UK	VR environments	Adults and children with intellectual disabilities (13)	Exploratory trials Focus groups
Wilson et al., 2019	Design/science & technology	Australia	An interactive ball	Autistic children (10)	Co-design beyond words
González et al., 2020	Education Architecture and design	Chile	A range of apps	Intellectual disabilities (10)	Double diamond method Design probes Group interviews Ideation: workshops User testing

Table 9.4   Overview of Hybrid Design studies

Study	Discipline	Country	Technology	User group	Tools & techniques
Russo et al., 2018	Computer science Robotics	Italy	Any	Mixed disabilities (9)	Hackability (UCD and PD)
Edler, 2020	Special education	Germany	Software	Cognitive disabilities	IPAR-UCD
Heumader et al., 2022	Computer science	Austria	Web-based AT recommender system	Cognitive disabilities (88)	IPAR-UCD

UCD Studies that Involved People with Disabilities

Five UCD studies were included in the review (Table 9.2). An example of a study that employed UCD is that conducted by Jie et al. (2020) who described their approach to redesigning the user interface of a sensor-feedback system for people recovering from stroke called 'Stappy'. The project was structured around the four phases of what is called the double diamond method: discovery, definition, development and delivery. The discovery phase established the user requirements through literature searches and data drawn from the related. In the definition phase, knowledge derived from the discovery phase was synthesised into a persona (an archetype of a user that is carefully described in terms of needs, goals and tasks). In the development and delivery phase, 15 participants with cognitive impairments and/or physical limitations were involved in iterative evaluations of prototypes.

PD Studies that Involved People with Disabilities

The review identified 14 PD studies (Table 9.3). An example of a study that employed PD is that conducted by Allin et al. (2018) who described their approach to involving people with spinal cord injury in the development of an online self-management program. The users were involved either as co-designers or as informants. Those operating as co-designers participated in daily design and prototyping meetings. Those operating as informants served as members of a Consumer Advisory Group which convened monthly.

Hybrid Studies that Involved People with Disabilities

When examining whether any studies adopted alternative approaches to UCD or PCD I identified three studies that could be considered hybrid in nature in that they were combining elements of two or more design approaches, at least one of which was either PD or UCD (Table 9.4). Russo et al. (2018: p. 158) describe Hackability as a method they have developed to enable makers, designers and people with disabilities to collaborate in order to solve specific problems that require customised solutions. They position Hackability as reflecting elements of both PD and UCD.

> It took 2 years to design the Hackability methodology to (i) increase the social inclusion of people with disabilities in the very same areas where they live, letting them work with makers on solving their specific needs following a *co-design* approach; (ii) let the makers focus their efforts considering the real needs expressed by people with disabilities, according to the User Center Design paradigm; (iii) develop a repository of ATs where solutions and devices are released Open Source to the community to be later implemented or improved.

Hackability has its origins in Hackathons and Makerspaces (Hatch, 2013) and essentially involves creating workgroups comprising people with disabilities and makers (designers). For each Hackability event, senior members of the Hackathon Association put out a call for 'needs' in order to recruit disabled participants and a call for skills in order to recruit makers. Two events are then organised. In the first event, disabled participants propose their specific technology need and makers describe their skill set. The makers and disabled participants then choose who they want to collaborate with and form workgroups. The workgroups then spend around a month coming up with their solution to the disabled person's need using an agile methodology (repeated and continued interaction with the disabled person). Each solution is then presented in a second closing event. The ultimate goal of a Hackability is to build strong relationships between local communities of makers and people with disabilities with the possibility of also fostering business opportunities.

Edler (2020) positions IPAR-UCD as a method that has been adapted from Inclusive Participatory Action Research and User-centred Design. Participatory Research (Cornwall & Jewkes, 1995), Participatory Action Research (Whyte, 1991), Inclusive Research (Walmsley & Johnson, 2003) and Inclusive Participatory Action Research (Ollerton, 2012) are a family of methods that involve people with disabilities as co-researchers or peer researchers. In combining IPAR and UCD, Edler (2020) argues that IPAR can be used to adapt and develop accessible methods and tools that enable the disabled person to be involved in the whole design process and that UCD can then be employed in the actual design of the technology. However, they provide no detail on how PAR was used to adapt the materials and methods, or on what the particular adaptations were. With regards to the UCD component of the method, Edler (2020) describes finding out about users' needs and requirements by asking the 'peer researchers' to try out different forms of support and assistance and then telling the developers what works well and what needs to be improved. This is then followed by iterative designing and redesigning involving a mix of methods that are used to promote the empowerment of the 'peer researchers', including focus groups, card sorting, scenarios, visual storytelling, cognitive walkthroughs and thinking aloud tests. Heumader et al. (2022) claim to be adopting IPAR-UCD, but they only describe the UCD component of designing an AT recommender system for users with cognitive disabilities – called Buddy. This component involved an end-user survey to determine how people with cognitive disabilities find, retrieve and use AT.

In the following sections I will critique each design approach in more detail.

What factors influence the choice of approach to involve users with disabilities in the design of AT?

The studies reporting the use of UCD were all conducted by research teams drawn from the disciplines of rehabilitation science, health sciences and engineering. There are, however, relatively few rehabilitation science and engineering research teams involved in PD or hybrid studies, suggesting that there may be disciplinary differences that influence the decisions that R&D teams make regarding which design approach to use when attempting to involve users with disabilities.

It is notable that none of the studies emanate from the Global South. Apart from this, the only discernible pattern relating to geography is that all of the hybrid studies and the majority of the PD studies are reported by European research teams. This is perhaps not surprising given that PD originates from Northern Europe. The PD, UCD and hybrid studies report developing a wide variety of technologies, from mobile apps and software to games and smart homes. This suggests that the type of technology being designed is not influencing how developers choose to involve users with disabilities.

The majority of UCD studies involved users with cognitive (dementia) and physical impairments, whereas the majority of PD and hybrid studies involved users with intellectual or learning disabilities. This is contrary to the findings of Seale et al. (2020) who observed that developers preferred not to use PD with users with learning disabilities. The mean size of user groups (when significant outliers such as the Layton et al., 2021 study are removed) is the same for both UCD and PD, around 19. Allin et al. (2018) note that a potential limitation of studies that employ participatory processes is that the generalisability of the end product may be limited. The extensive involvement of a relatively small group of users may result in a design that is tailored to only meet the needs of a small group.

What Justifications Are Given for the Choice of Approach for Involving People with Disabilities in the Design of Technologies?

The UCD studies did not explicitly reject PD or other approaches, but neither did they allocate a lot of space in their papers to explicitly justify UCD as a preferred approach. With the exception of Jie et al. (2020), it is not clear the UCD studies took the disability of their intended user into account when making their choices. The choice seems to be more influenced by the fact that studies involving similar technologies have used UCD. Jie et al. (2020) state that their overall goal was to create a meaningful user experience for people after stroke through designing a usable and enjoyable interface of the sensor-feedback system. To justify their use of UCD they draw parallels with patient involvement and other studies that have used UCD with users with cognitive disabilities. Richardson et al. (2021) offer no explicit rationale for their use of UCD over any other method. However, as their main objective was to assess the usability of their web-based app, it would seem a logical choice. The only literature they draw on to justify their choice was a study that also used UCD in the design of a patient information website. In a similar vein, Thirumalai et al. (2018) offer no explicit rationale for their choice of UCD and reference just one generic text on the principles of UCD. Grolier et al. (2023) justify their choice of UCD in order to maximise the effectiveness of the mobile app they were designing and reference two other studies that have used UCD to evaluable the usability of mobile apps. Ummels et al. (2022) claim that their UCD approach was an appropriate one to use in order to design a user-friendly interface and assess elderly people's use and experience of the adapted activity monitor in daily life. They cite two generic papers to support their case.

The majority of the PD studies did provide an explicit rationale for their use of PD as a design approach and cited a wide range of PD literature to support their case. Across the corpus of PD studies, seven reasons for using PD were offered: (1) to address the rights of people with disabilities; (2) because people with disabilities are experts in their own lives; (3) to focus on more than just the technical aspects of the design; (4) to provide a better design experience; (5)

to increase the quality of the final product; (6) to enhance the quality of life of the user; (7) to empower the user.

Both Layton et al. (2021) and Garcia et al. (2021) refer to the rights of people with disabilities to be co-creators in the design process. Layton et al. (2021: p. 1) argue that: "active co-design of AT services meets human rights and good practice benchmarks required by contemporary services". Wilson et al. (2019) and Williams and Gibson (2020) explain that they used PD because people with disabilities are experts in their own lives and therefore are best placed to shape the design of AT. Ferati et al. (2018: p. 248) explain that they used PD in order to focus on more than just the technical aspects of design. They wanted to "bridge the gap between a technical orientation and human-oriented approaches". Vollenwyder et al. (2020) talk about using PD in order to capture the subjective experience of users with disabilities. For Joshi and Valen (2018), PD provides a better design experience for users because it emphasises respect and inclusivity. Cosentino et al. (2021) suggest that people with disabilities can derive satisfaction and fun while feeling useful through their participation in a PD project.

Five PD studies argued that using this approach with users with disabilities would increase the quality of the final product (Aswad et al., 2022; Kortekaas & Zorn, 2022; Cosentino et al., 2021; Waardenburg et al., 2021; Allin et al., 2018). Indicators of quality included being accessible, non-stigmatising and effective. A key outcome of a producing a greater quality product through PD was suggested to be an increased likelihood of technology acceptance by the intended user group. One PD study argued that using PD methods would produce technologies that promote a better quality of life for users with disabilities (González et al., 2020).

Three studies justified the use of PD by arguing that it would empower the user (Harris et al., 2022; Waardenburg et al., 2021; Wilson et al., 2019). Wilson et al. (2019) argue that morality is a fundamental tenet of PD and that this morality is enacted by giving people with disabilities a say in design that affects their lives. Waardenburg et al. (2021) refer to the democratisation of innovation through the involvement of those who are typically marginalised in design. Given that involving users as equal partners in the design decisions is a core motivation for using the approach, it is perhaps surprising that not all the studies mentioned user empowerment as a core motivation for using PD with their disabled user groups. Furthermore, all of the studies were incredibly vague about how decisions were made in the PD teams and what specific decisions were made.

The stimulus for the creation of the Hackability approach by Russo et al. (2018) was an observation that people with disabilities often hack commercial devices or build custom solutions of their own in order to meet their needs. It must be noted that although the abstract refers to digital fabrication and customised joystick solutions, the two case studies presented in the main paper do not involve the 'making' of digital products, rather low-tech kitchen aids. Edler (2020) argues that they used IPAR-UCD because it caters for the needs of users with cognitive disabilities and therefore will increase the likelihood that the resulting software will be both usable and accepted by the intended user group. But Heumader et al. (2022) offers no explicit justification for employing IPAR-UCD.

Are the Approaches Adapted in Any Particular Way to Make Them More Accessible to People with Disabilities?

None of the UCD or hybrid studies explicitly mentioned adapting methods in any way for their users with disabilities. A handful of PD studies did report adapting their methods in order to facilitate communication or provide cognitive support (Harris et al., 2022; González et al., 2020; Williams & Gibson, 2020).

Harris et al. (2022) describe how they worked closely with teachers and support workers in order to facilitate communication with children and adults with intellectual impairments who were participating in their PD study. Williams and Gibson (2020) applied 'inclusive interviewing' techniques in order to facilitate the participation of people with learning disabilities in their PD project. This technique involved using short words, single-clause sentences, active verbs and the present tense when possible as well as avoiding abstract concepts and figurative or colloquial language. Wilson et al. (2019) describe how they merged practice-based methods drawn from speech and language therapy in order to facilitate communication with verbal children on the autism spectrum during the design process. These methods emphasised the need to recognise occurrences of 'in-the-moment' communicative actions such as joint attention, turn taking and imitation.

González et al. (2020) describe a raft of cognitive supports they used to facilitate the participation of people with intellectual impairment who were members of their Advisory Panel. In the preparation phase, such supports included using 'EasyRead' material in texts and presentations, in order to aid the understanding of concepts and procedures. In the fieldwork phase the designers adapted their design probe into a 'journey guide assistant'. For de-briefing and co-analysis they designed an elicitation log which enabled participants to produce a visual record of their experience. They also indicated that their users found it difficult to engage with unfinished prototypes such as wireframes which necessitated the use of more fully functional prototypes.

The observation that very few of the UCD and PD studies that I reviewed attempted to adapt their methods in order to make them accessible to their intended users with disabilities raises an important question about the extent to which people with disabilities were genuinely involved in the design process. If little or no attempts were made to ensure that the materials and activities used in the design process were adapted to meet the access needs of the users, there is the potential that user involvement was tokenistic rather than genuine.

Is there any evidence that one particular design approach is more effective at involving users with disabilities or produces more effective AT?

In seeking to examine whether one particular design approach is more effective at involving users with disabilities or produces more effective AT, I analysed what the studies had to say about both the benefits and challenges of employing their chosen design approach.

What Evaluative Evidence Is Provided to Demonstrate Successful Employment of the Approach with the Intended User Group?

All of the UCD and PD studies claimed that there were particular benefits to using their chosen design approach. However, they offered no detailed evidence to support their claim.

For example, Ummels et al. (2022) use the rather vague phrase 'swifter acceptance' as an indicator of the success of their UCD approach:

> This study contains several strengths and limitations that should be addressed. One strength of this study is its user-centred design [...] (early) involvement of the end-user is indispensable and offers several benefits, such as a swifter acceptance of the user interface, the capacity for users to identify problems specific to them, and the capacity for users to help define the scope of a project. (Ummels et al., 2022: p. 772)

In a similar vein, González et al. (2020: p. 62) make a rather sweeping claim that their PD approach has resulted in new, generalisable findings: "Including ID in codesign processes have proven of real value to general design knowledge. The incorporation of extreme users with special cognitive needs has resulted in new empirical knowledge that scales to other audiences through the optics of universal design."

Russo et al. (2018) claim that an indicator of the success of the Hackability method is that several municipalities recognised Hackability as an effective methodology to encourage social inclusion. No detailed evaluative evidence of the perceived success of the IPAR-UCD method was provided by Edler (2020) or Heumader et al. (2022).

What Challenges Are There in Employing Design Approaches with People with Disabilities?

It was noticeable that the UCD studies included in my review did not identify or discuss particular challenges related to involving people with disabilities in the design of technologies. Given that the PD studies were rather vague about how decisions were made and what decisions were made it is not surprising, although possibly disappointing, that none of them appear to have identified or discussed the possibility of co-designers within a team disagreeing with one another and how this issue might be managed to ensure the views of disabled co-designers are respected. For their hybrid IPAR-UCD study, Edler (2020: p. 47) did indicate that it can be challenging when the priorities of the disabled co-researchers are different from others in the team:

> Due to the complexity, attempts were made to solve the design requirements in a multidisciplinary way, often focusing less on technical issues and more on creativity. However, the latter proved to be a particular challenge. The peer researchers were primarily concerned with individual preferences in appearance and less with actual comprehensibility. However, standard design disciplines for product and communication design, as well as issues of ergonomics, information architecture, and usability research are important.

However, Edler (2020) offered no solution to the challenge. This could therefore be a useful focus for future research. Across the PD and hybrid studies capacity-related challenges for co-designers and co-researchers with and without disabilities were identified.

Capacity-related challenges for co-designers and co-researchers without disabilities

A key challenge for technology designers and researchers who involve people with disabilities in their design studies is having the skills and experience to communicate and interact with participants. The participants with disabilities are likely to have a vastly different lived experience and may also act and communicate in ways that are unfamiliar to designers and researchers without disabilities. Kortekaas and Zorn (2022) studied how an inexperienced researcher interacted with children with additional needs who lived in residential care. They noted that the communication strategies of this inexperienced and potentially nervous researcher closed discussions down in a way that was contradictory to the underlying aims of participatory design. In reflecting on the challenges of involving adults and children with intellectual disabilities, Harris et al. (2022) concluded that designers and researchers need to have prior experience of working with the group in order to be able build the kind of relationships required to facilitate detailed and meaningful feedback from disabled co-researchers. Kortekaas and Zorn (2022) propose that the challenge of inexperience can be addressed by pairing inexperienced researchers with more experienced researchers. They may also need to invest significant time visiting and getting to know the users with disabilities in the early phases of design studies, for example in the grant bidding or study design phases. This may help disabled co-designers to feel more confident and relaxed with the research team, which may facilitate communication of ideas and feedback later on in the study (Harris et al., 2022). Designers may also be able to gain experience of working with users with disabilities during their graduate training through internships or fieldwork.

Edler (2020) noted that it was a challenge to develop inclusive attitudes, procedures and methods so that the peer researchers were perceived as fully fledged members of the research team. Russo et al. (2018) shared that the co-design approach was sometimes misunderstood by makers in their Hackability events, leading them to take over or dominate in the workgroups. This suggests that, in addition to facilitating communication, capacity-building initiatives such as internships or fieldwork placements may also help to develop the inclusive attitudes that are required in order to perceive and treat disabled members of the design team as equal partners and to avoid them misunderstanding the intentions behind involving people with disabilities in the design process.

The experience reported by Kortekaas and Zorn (2022), Harris et al. (2022) and Edler (2020) reflect those of two studies conducted prior to 2018. Dekelver et al. (2015) and Allen et al. (2013) commented on the nature and the level of skills that researchers require in order to successfully engage in design projects with people with learning disability. Reflecting on their use of HCD, Dekelver et al. (2015) concluded that sociological skills were required in order to fully understand the specific position of people with learning disabilities at home and in care and work placement centres. Reflecting on their use of interactive sensory objects, Allen et al. (2013) reported that they had learnt the importance of using all their senses in order to give more chance of engagement to people with different disabilities and interests.

Capacity-related challenges for disabled co-designers and co-researchers

If people with disabilities are to be genuine partners in participatory design studies and operate on an equal basis with the developers/researchers, they need to have the skills or capacity required to understand and make decisions about the overall study and the design of the technology that is the focus of the study. This can be a particular challenge for people with cognitive disabilities or intellectual impairments. In reflecting on their participatory design study with adults with young autistic adults Waardenburg et al. (2021) suggested that the effectiveness of the participatory method will probably depend on the willingness and capacities of the users. In a similar vein, Williams and Gibson (2020) noted that particular care needs to be taken when co-designing with people with learning disabilities in terms of ensuring they understand the general aims of the study and the specific questions asked of them in each design phase.

Studies that are not underpinned by a PD philosophy tend to overcome the challenges related to cognitive capacity by engaging with proxies such as family, carers or expert professionals instead (see for example Gibson et al., 2019; Aakster et al., 2018). However, for studies that are committed to involving the user in the design of technologies, relying solely on proxies does not fully reflect the ideals of PD (or UCD for that matter). One current solution to this issue is to invite carers and professionals to support people with intellectual impairments or cognitive disabilities during the design process. An alternative, more empowering solution would be to invest in designing development opportunities that aim to build the capacity of people with disabilities to participate. One creative but rare example is that described by Boccardi et al. (2022) who developed a training programme modelled on the maker-space philosophy to enhance the knowledge of adults with intellectual and developmental disabilities regarding design processes and tools.

How can AT designers be supported to enhance the involvement of users with disabilities?

My review of UCD, PD and hybrid design studies suggests that the disability and technology community lacks a detailed shared understanding of why one approach may be preferable to another when attempting to increase user involvement in the design of technologies. It also appears to lack a shared commitment to undertaking a detailed evaluation of the successes and challenges of each design approach in order to inform future decision-making about how best to involve users with disabilities. This reflects the observations made by Stephens et al. (2023) and Kortekaas and Zorn (2022) in their critique of the PD field. This lack of evaluation and critical discussion, particularly of any failures or weaknesses in the employment of design approaches, may be symptomatic of the researchers' desire to show their work and product in a positive light in order to secure future funding. Nevertheless I would concur with Kortekaas and Zorn (2022) who argue that: "Current research in this area evidences a lack of systematic refection on and exploration or classification of methodological and research practice around the ambitions or assertions underlying and accompanying the establishment of participatory processes in technology development" (p. 311).

Furthermore, I would argue that there is a need for decision-making and evaluation frameworks to help support designers to effectively involve people with disabilities in the design of AT. In the following sections I will consider whether the foundations of such frameworks exist in the extant and related research literature.

Scoping the Potential Components of a Decision-making Framework

My review of design studies suggests that there may be three main factors that could influence whether designers choose PD, UCD or hybrid design approaches: the role or experience of the intended user group, the context or environment and available resources. For example, if the intended user group is one that is particularly marginalised or disadvantaged within society (e.g., learning disabilities/intellectual impairment) then there may be a particular emphasis on empowerment, which would suggest that PD would be an appropriate choice of design approach. Or if the designer/researcher has already decided on what kind of technology they want to design and has come up with some initial design ideas, then it may be more appropriate to employ UCD, which has less of an emphasis on the user being involved in all the key design decisions. With regards to context, if the proposed newly designed AT is intended to be used in health and social care settings, and its uptake is likely to be dependent on the recommendation or prescription of rehabilitation services, then UCD may be an appropriate choice of design approach, since there appears to be a close connection between the two (see Table 9.2). Similarly, if the key stakeholders (e.g., research funders or technology companies) have a preference for empirical data then UCD may be an appropriate choice because many standard usability tests are underpinned by empirical measurement. With regards to resources, if designers identify that they have sufficient time and expertise to build the capacity of users with disabilities and to involve them in all of the design stages including initial idea generation, then PD or hybrid design approaches may be appropriate.

These key design decisions reflect some of those suggested by Bühler (2000) and Draffan et al. (2016) who proposed frameworks for those aiming for the empowered participation of users with disabilities in technology-focused research and development projects. Bühler's framework, which he labels the 'FORTUNE concept,' is underpinned by seven principles: partnership as a basis; users are members of user organisations (so that they advocate on behalf of whole user group as well for themselves individually); the accessibility of all relevant materials and premises are guaranteed; every partner guarantees confidentiality, respect and expertise; there is a detailed plan for the project including time and resource planning for user participation; and partnership is implemented from the beginning of the project.

Draffan et al. (2016, p. 99) propose a framework to enable assistive technology designers to decide the level of participation that users with disabilities will be afforded with each design project (from non-involvement through to particimant initiated and directed). Their framework requires designers to consider the potential strengths of the user, the tasks required of the user, the resources required to enable participation (e.g., training) plus the expertise users bring with them, the environment in which they may be working and the tools they may need to support participation (e.g., communication aids). They argue that "careful analysis of all the components involved in the suggested framework can lead to better AT participatory design and research methodologies with potential users informing best practice".

Scoping the Potential Components of an Evaluation Framework

In scoping the potential components of an evaluation framework that might inform future decision-making about how best to involve users with disabilities, it may be helpful to explore the wider disability and technology literature. For example, I have identified three particular frameworks linked to participatory research. As part of the FORTUNE concept, Bühler (2001) offered a small checklist for evaluating user participation in projects. Researchers were asked to answer yes or no to questions such as:

1. Is the role and status of user participants clear?
2. Has user participation been formally authorised by user representatives?

3. Is there a budget for the labour, travel and personal assistants of the user participants?
4. Are all materials and premises accessible?
5. Does every partner guarantee confidentiality, respect and expertise?
6. Is there a detailed plan for the project including time, resources, ethics, safety, privacy and user benefit?
7. Is user partnership implemented before the project starts?

On its own, this checklist is probably too simplistic, and without expansion runs the risk of encouraging a 'tick-box' mentality, which is probably not appropriate in such a complex field.

One project that I was involved in used participatory research methods to involve people with intellectual and sensory impairments in the design of technologies to support inclusive museum experiences (Seale et al., 2021). We were unable to identify any existing frameworks for evaluating participatory design studies in the fields of inclusive museums, inclusive technologies or inclusive research in museums so we looked wider afield and identified a framework that had been used in health contexts. The International Collaboration for Participatory Health Research (ICPHR) has proposed a framework for evaluating the extent to which stakeholders are included in health research. ICPHR identified six concepts of validity in inclusive health research (see Table 9.5). We decided to try and apply this framework to our evaluation of the ARCHES project and developed a set of questions or issues that we felt reflected the six validities. We used a range of different data from different sources to answer these questions, including stakeholder and user interviews, field notes, i-poems and body-mapping. There is some similarity between this framework and that offered by Bühler in relation to the emphasis on the role and status of users and on ethical practice.

In Chapter 3 of this book, Alan Foley explains how he used a framework derived from the principles of Participatory Action Research to evaluate the success of a technology design project involving users with intellectual impairments. The four evaluation questions were:

1. Did people with disabilities articulate the problem and participate directly in the process?
2. Did direct involvement of people with disabilities in the research process allow participants to share objective and subjective aspects of their (lived) experience?

Table 9.5   Application of the ICHPR's six validities to evaluating design studies that seek to involve users with disabilities

Validity	Applied to design project	Example questions
Participatory validity	Does the design project allow participants to play a full and active part in the design process?	Who took part in each activity and who did not? How were decisions taken within the group? Were any decisions or activities blocked within the group, if so, why? If not, what reasons were given? Did participants understand that the project was meant to be participatory? Were there any signs or occasions where participants appeared confused and unsure about the participatory nature of the project or seemed to positively embrace or reject the participatory nature of the project? How were participants supported to understand and enact design practices?
Intersubjective validity	Is the design project credible and meaningful to participants?	Did the participants recognise and value what the project is trying to achieve?
Contextual validity	Is the design project relevant to the local situation (i.e., sensitive to the needs, interests and motivations of individuals in the group)?	Was the design project relevant to participants' needs and interests? Have the participants' motivations for joining the project been realised?
Catalytic validity	Is the design project creating opportunities for change or action?	Have things changed because of participants' involvement in the project? If so, what? Was the change (actual or potential) within the project or beyond the project?
Ethical validity	Is the design project sound and just in what it is trying to achieve and the way it is trying to achieve it?	Was the project managed in a fair way? Were participants fairly treated? Were all members of the group treated in an equal way?
Empathetic validity	Is the design project increasing empathy among participants?	Did all participants (including designers) come to understand the perspectives of others involved across the project? Did all participants (including users with disabilities) feel part of a community/team/group?

3. Did participating in PAR increase awareness among the disabled participants about their own resources and strengths and help develop leadership
   skills among the participants?
4. Did the PAR project improve the quality of life for people with disabilities?

The focus on articulating the problem and participating directly in the process
reflects the first and seventh questions in Bühler's evaluation framework and
also resonates with the concept of participatory validity. The focus on increasing awareness of disabled participants and improving their quality of life has
similarities with the concept of catalytic validity.

There may be potential for the validities and questions identified across the
three frameworks to be adapted to the evaluation of future design studies that
seek to involve users with disabilities. However, further research is needed
to assess the extent to which they are applicable to those design approaches
that are not underpinned by participatory design or research principles. In
addition, the three frameworks that I have reviewed focus on the process of
design and not the outcomes of the design process. Therefore, answering these
questions may tell us whether users with disabilities have had a good design
experience, but it may not necessarily tell us whether the resulting technology
is any 'better' than those that have been designed without involving people
with disabilities.

Conclusions: What are the implications for a future research agenda?

In this chapter I have reported on the results of a critical review of studies
reporting to involve people with disabilities in the design of new technologies.
The majority of the studies used either UCD or PD approaches to involve
people with disabilities. The choice of these approaches did not appear to be
linked to the particular disability of the user group, or the particular technology being designed. It was not common practice for design studies to provide
an explicit justification for their choice of design approach or to adapt their
design tools and techniques to make them more accessible to disabled participants. There was also a general lack of detailed evaluations of the success of the
design approaches. The most commonly identified challenge was related to the
design skills and experience of both designers and participants. These results
have a number of implications for a future research agenda.

Firstly, it is important for future research and development studies that involve people with disabilities to provide a much more detailed justification for their choice of design approach and to make their decision-making process more explicit. Secondly, future research could make a significant contribution to the field by developing and evaluating appropriate and successful methods for building the capacity of designers and developers to meaningfully involve users with disabilities. The development and evaluation of a wider range of capacity-building activities and resources for people with disabilities could also be a valuable addition to a future research agenda. There is also a need to develop detailed decision-making and evaluation frameworks that have the potential to help designers to effectively involve people with disabilities in the design of AT.

It is important to acknowledge that the studies reviewed in this chapter focused solely on involving people with disabilities in the process of designing technologies that are oriented specifically towards meeting their needs. In order to contribute to current debates surrounding the mainstreaming of technologies and the practicalities of Universal Design, future research could usefully evaluate the extent to which people with disabilities and people without disabilities can collaborate in the technology design process to produce new technologies that meet the needs of both groups. The starting point for such design studies might be UCD and PD, but the end point could be a completely new approach to involving users in the design of technologies.

References

Aakster, Y., van Delden, R., & Lentelink, S. (2018). Lost Puppy: Towards a Playful Intervention for Wandering Dementia Patients. In A. Cheok, A. Inami, & M. Romão (Eds.), *Advances in Computer Entertainment Technology. ACE 2017. Lecture Notes in Computer Science, vol 10714* (pp. 84–102). Springer. https://doi.org/10.1007/978-3-319-76270-8_7

Abras, C., Maloney-Krichmar, D., & Preece, J. (2004). User-Centered Design. In W. Bainbridge (Ed.), *Encyclopedia of Human-Computer Interaction* (pp. 445–456). Thousand Oaks.

Allen, K., Hollinworth, N., Minnion, A., Kwiatkowska, G., Lowe, T., Weldin, N., & Hwang, F. (2013). Interactive sensory objects for improving access to heritage. *Proceedings of CHI '13 Extended Abstracts on Human Factors in Computing Systems (CHI EA '13)* (pp. 2899–2902). Association for Computing Machinery. https://doi.org/10.1145/2468356.2479569

Allin, S., Shepherd, J., Tomasone, J., Munce, S., Linassi, G., Hossain, S.N., & Jaglal, S. (2018). Participatory design of an online self-management tool for users with spinal cord injury: Qualitative study. *JMIR Rehabilitation and Assistive Technologies*, 5(1):e6. https://rehab.jmir.org/2018/1/e6/

Aswad, E., Murphy, E., Fernandez-Rivera, C., & Boland, S. (2022). Towards an Inclusive Co-design Toolkit: Perceptions and Experiences of Co-design Stakeholders. In K. Miesenberger, G. Kouroupetroglou, K. Mavrou, R. Manduchi, R.M. Covarrubias, & P. Penáz (Eds.), *Computers Helping People with Special Needs. ICCHP-AAATE 2022. Lecture Notes in Computer Science, vol 13342* (pp. 284–292). Springer. https://doi.org/10.1007/978-3-031-08645-8_33

Blomberg, J.L., & Henderson, A. (1990). Reflections on participatory design: Lessons from the trillium experience. *Proceedings of the SIGCHI Conference on Human Factors in Computing Systems CHI '90 (pp. 353).* Association for Computing Machinery. https://doi.org/10.1145/97243.97307

Boccardi, A., Szucs, K.A., Ebuenyi, I.D., & Mhatre, A. (2022). Assistive technology makerspaces promote capability of adults with intellectual and developmental disabilities. *Societies, 12*(6), 155. https://doi.org/10.3390/soc12060155

Bødker, S., Grønbaek, K., & Kyng, M. (1993). Cooperative Design: Techniques and Experiences from the Scandinavian Scene. In D. Schuler & A. Namioka (Eds.), *Participatory Design: Principles and Practices* (1st edition, pp. 157–175). CRC Press. https://doi.org/10.1201/9780203744338

Bühler, C. (2001). Empowered participation of users with disabilities in R&D projects. *International Journal of. Human-Computer Studies, 55*(4), 645–659 https://doi.org/10.1006/ijhc.2001.0489

Carroll, J.M., Chin, G., Rosson, M.B., & Neale, D.C. (2000). The development of cooperation: Five years of participatory design in the virtual school. *Proceedings of the 3rd Conference on Designing Interactive Systems: Processes, Practices, Methods, and Techniques (DIS '00)* (pp. 239–251). Association for Computing Machinery. https://doi.org/10.1145/347642.347731

Cornwall, A., & Jewkes, R. (1995). What is participatory research? *Social Science and Medicine, 41*(12), 1667–1676. DOI:10.1016/0277–9536(95)00127-s

Cosentino, G., Morra, D., Gelsomini, M., Matera, M., & Mores, M. (2021). COBO: A Card-Based Toolkit for Co-Designing Smart Outdoor Experiences with People with Intellectual Disability. In C. Ardito, R. Lanzilotti, A. Malizia, H. Petrie, A. Piccinno, G. Desolda, & Inkpen, K. (Eds.), *Human-Computer Interaction – INTERACT 2021. Lecture Notes in Computer Science, vol 12932* (pp. 149–169). Springer. https://doi.org/10.1007/978-3-030-85623-6_11

Dekelver, J., Daems, J., Solberg, S., Bosch, N., Van De Perre, L., & De Vliegher, A. (2015). Viamigo: A digital travel assistant for people with intellectual disabilities: Modelling and design using contemporary intelligent technologies as a support for independent traveling of people with intellectual disabilities. *Proceedings of 6th International Conference on Information, Intelligence, Systems and Applications* (pp. 1–6). IEEE. DOI:10.1109/IISA.2015.7388014

Dirks, S. (2019). Empowering Instead of Hindering – Challenges in Participatory Development of Cognitively Accessible Software. In M. Antona & C. Stephanidis (Eds.), *Universal Access in Human-Computer Interaction. Theory, Methods and Tools. HCII 2019. Lecture Notes in Computer Science, vol 11572* (pp. 28–38). Springer. https://doi.org/10.1007/978-3-030-23560-4_3

Draffan, E.A., James, A., Wald, M., & Idris, A. (2016). Framework for selecting assistive technology user-participation methods. *Journal of Assistive Technologies, 10*(2), 92–101. https://doi.org/10.1108/JAT-01-2016-0007

Edler, C.M.A. (2020). IPAR-UCD – Inclusive Participation of Users with Cognitive Disabilities in Software Development. In K. Miesenberger, G. Kouroupetroglou, K. Mavrou, R. Manduchi, R.M. Covarrubias, & P. Penáz (Eds.), *Computers Helping People with Special Needs. ICCHP 2020. Lecture Notes in Computer Science, vol 12376* (pp. 43–50). https://doi.org/10.1007/978-3-030-58796-3_6

Ellis, R.D., & Kurniawan, S. (2000). Increasing the usability of online information for older users: A case study in participatory design. *International Journal of Human-Computer Interaction, 12*(2), 263–276. https://doi.org/10.1207/S15327590IJHC1202_6

Ferati, M., Babar, A., Carine, K., Hamidi, A., & Mörtberg, C. (2018). Participatory Design Approach to Internet of Things: Co-designing a Smart Shower for and with People with Disabilities. In M. Antona & C. Stephanidis (Eds.), *Universal Access in Human-Computer Interaction. Virtual, Augmented, and Intelligent Environments, UAHCI 2018. Lecture Notes in Computer Science, vol 10908* (pp. 246–261). Springer-Verlag. https://doi.org/10.1007/978-3-319-92052-8_19

Garcia, L.S., Felipe, T.A., Guedes, A.P., Antunes, D.R., Iatskiu, C.E., Todt, E., Bueno, J., Trindade, D.F.G., Gonçalves, D.A., Canteri, R., Canal, M.C., Ferreira, M.A.M., Silva, A.M.C., Galvão, L., & Rodrigues, L. (2021). Deaf Inclusion Through Brazilian Sign Language: A Computational Architecture Supporting Artifacts and Interactive Applications and Tools. In M. Antona & C. Stephanidis (Eds.), *Universal Access in Human-Computer Interaction. Access to Media, Learning and Assistive Environments. HCII 2021. Lecture Notes in Computer Science, vol 12769* (pp. 167–185). Springer. https://doi.org/10.1007/978-3-030-78095-1_14

Gibson, R.C., Bouamrane, M.M., & Dunlop, M. (2019). Design requirements for a digital aid to support adults with mild learning disabilities during clinical consultations: Qualitative study with experts. *JMIR Rehabilitation & Assistive Technologies, 6*(1): e10449. DOI:10.2196/10449

González, H.S., Córdova, V.V., Cid, K.E., Azagra, M.J., & Alvarez-Aguado, I. (2020). Including intellectual disability in participatory design processes: Methodological adaptations and supports. *Proceedings of the 16th Participatory Design Conference 2020 – Participation(s) Otherwise* (vol. 1, pp. 55–63). https:// doi .org/ 10 .1145/ 3385010.3385023

Gould, J., & Lewis, C. (1985). Designing for usability: Key principles and what designers think. *Communications of the ACM, 28*(3), 300–311. DOI:10.1145/3166.3170

Greenbaum, J., & Kyng, M. (1991). *Design at Work: Cooperative Design of Computer Systems.* Lawrence Erlbaum Associates.

Grolier, M., Arefyev, A., Pereira, B., Figueiredo, I.T., Gerbaud, L., & Coudeyre, E. (2023). Refining the design of a smartphone application for people with chronic low back pain using mixed quantitative and qualitative approaches. *Disability and Rehabilitation: Assistive Technology, 18*(2), 145–150. DOI:10.1080/17483107.2020. 1839575

Harris, M.C., Brown, D.J., Vyas, P., & Lewis, J. (2022). A Methodology for the Co-design of Shared VR Environments with People with Intellectual Disabilities: Insights from the Preparation Phase. In M. Antona & C. Stephanidis (Eds.), *Universal Access in Human-Computer Interaction. User and Context Diversity. HCII 2022. Lecture Notes in Computer Science, vol 13309* (pp. 217–230). Springer. https:// doi .org/ 10 .1007/978-3-031-05039-8_15

Hatch, M. (2013). *The Maker Movement Manifesto: Rules for Innovation in the New World of Crafters, Hackers, and Tinkerers.* McGraw Hill Professional.

Heumader, P., Murillo-Morales, T., & Miesenberger, K. (2022). Buddy – A Personal Companion to Match People with Cognitive Disabilities and AT. In K. Miesenberger,

G. Kouroupetroglou, K. Mavrou, R. Manduchi, R.M. Covarrubias, & P. Penáz (Eds.), *Computers Helping People with Special Needs. ICCHP-AAATE 2022. Lecture Notes in Computer Science, vol 13342* (pp. 275–283). Springer. https://doi.org/10.1007/978-3-031-08645-8_32

Jie, L-J., Jamin, G., Smit, K., Beurskens, A., & Braun, S. (2020). Design of the user interface for 'Stappy', a sensor-feedback system to facilitate walking in people after stroke: A user-centred approach. *Disability and Rehabilitation: Assistive Technology, 15*(8), 959–967. DOI:10.1080/17483107.2019.1629654

Joshi, S.G., & Valen, J. (2018). Co-exploring Interaction Opportunities for Enabling Technologies for People with Rheumatic Disorder. In K. Miesenberger & G. Kouroupetroglou (Eds.), *Computers Helping People with Special Needs. ICCHP 2018. Lecture Notes in Computer Science, vol 10896* (pp. 415–523) Springer. https://doi.org/10.1007/978-3-319-94277-3_65

Kensing, F., & Blomberg, J. (1998). Participatory design: Issues and concerns. *Computer Supported Cooperative Work, 7*, 167–185. https://doi.org/10.1023/A:1008689307411

Kortekaas, C., & Zorn, I. (2022). Communication Styles as Challenges for Participatory Design Process Facilitators Working with Young People with Additional Needs in a Residential Care Setting: A Conversation Analysis. In K. Miesenberger, G. Kouroupetroglou, K. Mavrou, R. Manduchi, R.M. Covarrubias, & P. Penáz (Eds.), *Computers Helping People with Special Needs. ICCHP-AAATE 2022. Lecture Notes in Computer Science, vol 13342* (pp. 310–319). Springer. https://doi.org/10.1007/978-3-031-08645-8_36

Layton, N., Harper, K., Martinez, K., Berrick, N., & Naseri, C. (2021). Co-creating an assistive technology peer-support community: Learnings from AT Chat. *Disability and Rehabilitation: Assistive Technology, 18*(5), 603–609. DOI:10.1080/17483107.2021.1897694

Mao, J.-Y., Vredenburg, K., Smith, P.W., & Carey, T. (2005). The state of user-centred design practice. *Communications of the ACM, 48*(3), 105–109. https://doi.org/10.1145/1047671.1047677

Muller, M.J., & Druin, A. (2012). Participatory Design: The Third Space in Human-Computer Interaction. In J.A. Jacko (Ed.), *Human Computer Interaction Handbook: Fundamentals, Evolving Technologies, and Emerging Applications* (3rd edition, pp. 1125–1153). Taylor & Francis Group.

Muller, M.J., Haslwanter, J.H., & Dayton, T. (1997). Participatory Practices in the Software Lifecycle. In M. Helander, T.K. Landauer, & P. Prabhu (Eds.), *Handbook of Human-Computer Interaction* (2nd edition, pp. 255–297). Elsevier.

Muller, M.J., & Kuhn, S. (1993). Participatory design. *Communications of the ACM, 36*(6), 24–28. https://doi.org/10.1145/153571.255960

Nelson, J., Buisine, S., & Aoussat, A. (2013). Anticipating the use of future things: Towards a framework for prospective use analysis in innovation design projects. *Applied Ergonomics, 44*(6), 948–956. https://doi.org/10.1016/j.apergo.2013.01.002

Newell, A.F., Gregor, P., Morgan, M., Pullin, G., & Macaulay, C. (2011). User-sensitive inclusive design. *Universal Access in the Information Society, 10*(3), 235–243. https://doi.org/10.1007/s10209-010-0203-y

Ollerton, J.M. (2012). IPAR, an inclusive disability research methodology with accessible analytical tools. *International Practice Development Journal, 2*(2), [3]. https://www.fons.org/Resources/Documents/Journal/Vol2No2/IPDJ_0202_03.pdf

Preece, J.J., Rogers, Y.R., Sharp, H., Benyon, D.R., Holland, S., & Carey, T. (1994). *Human-Computer Interaction.* Addison-Wesley.

Richardson, J., Letts, L., Sinclair, S., Chan, D., Miller, J., Donnelly, C., Smith-Turchyn, J., Wojkowski, S., Gravesande, J., & Sánchez, A.L. (2021). Using a web-based app to deliver rehabilitation strategies to persons with chronic conditions: Development and usability study. *JMIR Rehabilitation & Assistive Technologies*, 8(1):e19519. DOI:10.2196/19519

Russo, L.O., Airò Farulla, G., & Boccazzi Varotto, C. (2018). Hackability: A Methodology to Encourage the Development of DIY Assistive Devices. In K. Miesenberger & G. Kouroupetroglou (Eds.), *Computers Helping People with Special Needs. ICCHP 2018. Lecture Notes in Computer Science, vol 10897* (pp. 156–163). Springer. https://doi.org/10.1007/978-3-319-94274-2_22

Sanders, E.B.N., Brandt, E., & Binder, T. (2010). A framework for organizing the tools and techniques of participatory design. *Proceedings of the 11th Biennial Participatory Design Conference (PDC '10)* (pp. 195–198). Association for Computing Machinery. https://doi.org/10.1145/1900441.1900476

Sanders, E.B.N., & Stappers, P.J. (2008). Co-creation and the new landscapes of design. *CoDesign: International Journal of CoCreation in Design and the Arts*, 4(1), 5–18. https://doi.org/10.1080/15710880701875068

Seale, J., Carrizosa, H.G., Rix, J., Sheehy, K., & Hayhoe, S. (2021). A participatory approach to the evaluation of participatory museum research projects. *International Journal of Research and Method in Education*, 44(1), 20–40. https://doi.org/10.1080/1743727X.2019.1706468

Seale, J., Carrizosa, H.G., Rix, J., Sheehy, K., & Hayhoe, S. (2020). In Search of a Decision-Making Framework for Involving Users Who Have Learning Disabilities or Sensory Impairments in the Process of Designing Future Technologies. In K. Aria, R. Bhatia, & S. Kapoor (Eds.), *Proceedings of the Future Technologies Conference (FTC) 2019. Advances in Intelligent Systems and Computing, vol 1069* (pp. 844–861). Springer. https://doi.org/10.1007/978-3-030-32520-6_61

Stephens, L., Smith, H., Epstein, I., Baljko, M., Mcintosh,I., Dadashi, N., & Prakash, D.N. (2023). Accessibility and participatory design: Time, power, and facilitation. *CoDesign*. DOI:10.1080/15710882.2023.2214145

Thirumalai, M., Kirkland, W.B., Misko, S.R., Padalabalanarayanan, S., & Malone, L.A. (2018). Adapting the Wii Fit balance board to enable active video game play by wheelchair users: User-centered design and usability evaluation. *JMIR Rehabilitation & Assistive Technologies*, 5(1):e2. DOI:10.2196/rehab.8003

Travnicek, C., Stoll, D., Reichinger, A., & Rix, J. (2022). It soon became clear – insights into technology and participation. *Qualitative Research Journal*, 22(2), 129–142. https://doi.org/10.1108/QRJ-03-2021-0035

Ummels, D., Braun, S., Stevens, A., Beekman, E., & Beurskens, A. (2022). Measure It Super Simple (MISS) activity tracker: (re)Design of a user-friendly interface and evaluation of experiences in daily life. *Disability and Rehabilitation: Assistive Technology*, 17(7), 767–777. DOI:10.1080/17483107.2020.1815089

Vollenwyder, B., Buchmüller, E., Trachsel, C., Opwis, K., & Brühlmann, F. (2020). My Train Talks to Me: Participatory Design of a Mobile App for Travellers with Visual Impairments. In K. Miesenberger, G. Kouroupetroglou, K. Mavrou, R. Manduchi, R.M. Covarrubias, & P. Penáz (Eds.), *Computers Helping People with Special Needs. ICCHP 2020. Lecture Notes in Computer Science, vol 12376* (pp. 10–18). Springer. https://doi.org/10.1007/978-3-030-58796-3_2

Waardenburg, T., van Huizen, N., van Dijk, J., Mangée, M., Staal, W., Teunisse, J-P., & van der Voort, M. (2021). Design Your Life: User-Initiated Design of Technology to Support Independent Living of Young Autistic Adults. In M.M. Soares, E.

Rosenwieg, & A. Marcus (Eds.), *Design, User Experience, and Usability: Design for Diversity, Well-being, and Social Development. HCII 2021. Lecture Notes in Computer Science, vol 12780* (pp. 373–386). Springer. https://doi.org/10.1007/978-3-030-78224-5_26

Walmsley, J., & Johnson, K. (2003). *Inclusive Research with People with Learning Disabilities*. Jessica Kingsley Publishers.

Whyte, W.F. (1991). *Participatory Action Research*. Sage Publications.

Williams, P., & Gibson, P. (2020). CVT connect: Creating safe and accessible social media for people with learning disabilities. *Technology and Disability, 32*(2), 81–92. DOI:10.3233/TAD-200259

Wilson, C., Brereton, M., Ploderer, B., & Sitbon, L. (2019). Co-design beyond words: 'Moments of interaction' with minimally-verbal children on the autism spectrum. *Proceedings of the 2019 CHI Conference on Human Factors in Computing Systems* (pp. 1–15). ACM. https://doi.org/10.1145/3290605.3300251

10. Addressing the main challenges of future assistive technology research by building a community of practice

Jane Seale

Introduction

In Chapters 1 and 2 of this book I argued that there were five main challenges that future research in the field of disability and technology needs to address:

1. Addressing the impact that different conceptions of disability and technology can have on assistive technology (AT) research and development
2. Finding solutions that address the complexity of digital inequalities
3. Developing meaningful and comprehensive methods for capturing and evaluating the outcomes of AT use
4. Understanding the history of AT in order to imagine the future of AT
5. Increasing the involvement of people with disabilities in the design and development of new technologies

In different ways and in different contexts each contributing chapter of this edited book has endorsed one or more of these challenges. With regards to the impact of different conceptions of disability, in Chapter 3, Alan Foley suggests that many academic research institutions have an ableist culture which will limit the extent to which academic researchers can meaningfully involve people with disabilities in the design and development of new technologies. With regards to conceptions of technology, in Chapter 5, Gregg Vanderheiden, Crystal Marte and J. Bern Jordan outline a proposal to develop a new technology that combines an Info-Bot with an Individual User Interface Generator (IUIG). This proposal is built on two alternative conceptualisations of technology: firstly, that technology adapts to the user's needs, rather than requiring the user to adapt to the technology because it addresses their specific accessibility needs; and secondly, that new technologies can augment rather than replace existing or more traditional technologies.

A number of chapters offered potential solutions to addressing the complexity of digital inequalities. In Chapter 4, Paul Whittington and Huseyin Dogan proposed solutions to challenges that people with disabilities experience when required to authenticate themselves or communicate their accessibility requirements through traditional methods. In Chapter 5, Gregg Vanderheiden, Crystal Marte and J. Bern Jordan argued that an alternate approach to accessibility is required in order to fill the growing gap of products that people need access to, but do not have accommodations for. In Chapter 8, Rohan Slaughter, Annalu Waller and Tom Griffiths argue that in order to increase the number of people with disabilities who can benefit from using AT we need more trained, professional Assistive Technologists who can support and adapt the use of AT to meet the needs of people with disabilities in a range of settings.

Chapters 6 and 7 offered some insights into the challenge of capturing and evaluating the outcomes of AT use. In Chapter 6, Robert McLaren, Shamima Akhtar and Clive Gilbert focused on how policy makers need evidence and data regarding AT outcomes and impact in order to inform AT policy decisions about the funding and delivery of AT and AT services. They suggest that researchers need to make this information more discoverable and that broader-based research (e.g., systematic reviews and meta-analyses) is required. In Chapter 7, Dave Edyburn pointed to the potential for imminent advances in machine learning and artificial intelligence to improve the evidencing of outcomes of AT use.

In mapping out their visions for the future of AT and AT research, several chapter authors contextualised and explained their vision by providing a history of their field. For example, in Chapter 5, in order to make a case for an alternate supplemental approach to traditional approaches to accessibility, Gregg Vanderheiden, Crystal Marte and J. Bern Jordan recounted the evolution of ICT accessibility from the 1960s onwards. In Chapter 7, Dave Edyburn offered a history of policy, innovative product development and research over the last 40 years in order to illuminate drivers for change. In Chapter 8, as part of building their case for the professionalisation of Assistive Technologists, Rohan Slaughter, Annalu Waller and Tom Griffiths discussed past initiatives and identified strengths or successes that can inform a future vision for training and capacity-building in the field.

In Chapters 3 and 9, Alan Foley and I discussed and evaluated different methods for increasing the involvement of people with disabilities in the design and development of new technologies. In Chapter 3, Alan Foley proposed Participatory Action Research as a method that has the potential to involve one of the most marginalised disability groups in the field, people with intellectual disabilities. In Chapter 9, I examined the extent to which a shared understanding exists in the disability and technology community regarding what greater 'user involvement' means and how to achieve it.

In mapping ways forward in meeting these and other challenges of future research in the field, suggestions by the chapter authors fell into two interconnected categories: 1) a call for greater interdisciplinarity and 2) a call to build different, collaborative relationships with stakeholders in the field. In Chapter 7, Dave Edyburn encouraged readers to engage in interdisciplinary conversations that have the potential to dramatically alter the provision and use of AT. In Chapter 8, the authors made a case for undertaking interdisciplinary research that seeks to evidence the impact of dedicated AT roles.

With regards to building different relationships, Gregg Vanderheiden, Crystal Marte and J. Bern Jordan suggested that their proposed new technology comprising an Info-Bot and IUIG will require a different working relationship or social contract between product developers and AT users. In Chapter 6, Robert McLaren, Shamima Akhtar and Clive Gilbert argued that there needs to be better connections between policy makers and researchers so that government AT-related policy is underpinned by a broader evidence base. The authors of Chapters 7 and 8 called for greater collaboration between all the AT stakeholders. Dave Edyburn argued for more practice-inspired collaborative research that includes users. He also encouraged "individuals and groups to propose, disseminate, and critique proposed research agendas in order to spark conversation, debate, and collaboration about the future of AT research". Rohan Slaughter, Annalu Waller and Tom Griffiths called on a range of stakeholders including AT users, academic researchers and health and social care practitioners to support their capacity-building and research efforts.

The calls for building more interdisciplinary and/or collaborative relationships from our chapter authors echo calls from the community at large. For example, the World Health Organization (WHO) and United Nations Children's Fund (UNICEF) call for greater collaboration between professions responsible for AT service provision:

> Assistive technology should not be regarded as under the control of any single profession. As it becomes more widely used, and increasingly overlaps with digital technologies, assistive technology will become a necessary competence for all professions involved in service provision for persons with disabilities, older people,

those living with chronic conditions including mental health conditions, etc. This means that policy should encourage governance models that promote open, interdisciplinary and collaborative approaches to decision-making, both across disciplines and with users being centrally engaged in joint decision-making. Good governance promotes effective interdisciplinary working by explicitly designing how interdependencies among individuals, groups and sectors should be promoted, developed and maintained in order to deliver cost-effective integrated services. (WHO & UNICEF, 2022, p. 70)

Others call for greater collaboration between researchers and practitioners. For example, Pascher et al. (2021) suggest that collaboration is beneficial because researchers can focus on the technical aspects and practitioners can focus on the social aspects. For others, collaboration is understood more broadly as involving researchers/academics, technology developers, professionals, caregivers and users (e.g., Van den Heuvel et al., 2022). In August 2023, at a roundtable discussion on the way forward and priorities for the global AT agenda, Evert-Jan Hoogerwerf, Secretary-General of the Association for the Advancement of Assistive Technology in Europe (AAATE), proposed that we need a community of researchers, users, practitioners and researchers. He called for the creation of an eco-system, moving forward together towards the policy level, where changes need to be made.[1]

This chapter will examine in more detail how the field of disability and technology currently understands interdisciplinarity, potential barriers to developing interdisciplinary research and how the field can build capacity to conduct effective interdisciplinary research in the future.

Definitions and understandings of what constitutes interdisciplinary research in the AT field

In the generic (i.e., not focused specifically on AT) literature that spans disciplines such as science, technology, health and business, interdisciplinarity is broadly understood as involving the integration of discrete separate bodies of knowledge with each other in order to create new knowledge (Cheng et al., 2009; Aboelela et al., 2007; Tait & Lyall, 2007; Griffin et al., 2006; Institute of Medicine, 2005):

> Interdisciplinary research is a mode of research by teams or individuals that *integrates* information, data, techniques, tools, perspectives, concepts, and/or theories from two or more disciplines or bodies of specialized knowledge to advance fundamental understanding or to solve problems whose solutions are *beyond the scope of a single discipline* or area of research practice. (Institute of Medicine, 2005, p. 2)

Klein and Newell (1997) define interdisciplinary work as combining the expertise of one or more disciplines to find a solution to a complex problem. Tait and Lyall (2007) state that the setting up and funding of interdisciplinary research programmes is motivated by desires to transfer information from the laboratory to the real world, to be user-driven and to be relevant to policy making in complex areas. Tait and Lyall (2007) and Griffin et al. (2006) also argue that there are two different types of interdisciplinary research that can be distinguished based on their overarching aims or knowledge seeking strategies:

1. Research which aims to further the expertise and competence of academic disciplines themselves, e.g., through developments in methodology which enable new issues to be addressed or new disciplines or sub-disciplines to be formed (discipline-focused)
2. Research which is problem-focused and addresses issues of social, technical and/or policy relevance with less emphasis on discipline-related academic outcomes (problem-focused)

Smith and Boger (2022) argue that AT provision is inherently interdisciplinary because addressing people's AT needs requires a coordinated and sustained collaboration between people with clinical and technical expertise as well as AT users. Consequently, it is therefore natural for AT research to be equally interdisciplinary, drawing on the skills and knowledge of practitioners, engineers, service providers and others in order to innovative approaches and new ways of thinking. However, my review of the AT literature suggests that there is not a standard or shared understanding of what interdisciplinary research means or looks like. For example, some literature uses the term 'interdisciplinary' interchangeably with terms such as 'multidisciplinary' (see for example Koumpouros, 2021). Other studies position AT research as either a collaboration between different academic disciplines, a collaboration between academics and practitioners or a multistakeholder collaboration that includes users. Furthermore, there is a small but growing group of AT researchers who are calling for transdisciplinary rather than interdisciplinary research.

Understanding Interdisciplinarity as Collaboration between Different Academic Disciplines

A range of researchers indicate that mixing disciplines is necessary in their specific area of AT research. For example, Haltaufderheide et al. (2020) propose that mixing the disciplines of nursing science, social sciences, philosophy, medical ethics, economics and law is needed in order to examine the implications of using socially assistive technologies in health care. Plattner et al. (2020) argue that in the field of smart homes and smart care for the elderly, it is important to focus on both the technical and human aspects, which requires people from the technical field to work together with sociologists, economists or medical scientists in collaborative projects to develop and offer these services. Schwaninger et al. (2021) claim that empirical research in human–robot interaction requires interdisciplinary teams comprising gerontologists, social scientists and engineers, while Shaw et al. (2022) contend that the complex nature of using a child-centred approach for designing wheelchairs requires collaboration between academics with expertise in inclusive paediatric mobility (IPM) design, inclusive design and children's rights and disability.

Understanding Interdisciplinarity as Collaboration between Practitioners and Academics

A small but influential core of AT research, particularly that conducted in health and rehabilitative settings, understands interdisciplinarity as the mixing of academic researchers with clinical or rehabilitation practitioners. For example, writing in the context of the ageing and technology agenda, Schulz et al. (2015, p. 731) argue that:

> Successful technology development requires unprecedented interdisciplinary collaboration. As gerontologists, we are accustomed to working in interdisciplinary teams, but the development of successful technology requires teams that not only include clinicians, social and behavioral scientists, and policy experts but also include engineers, human factors specialists, computer scientists, designers, and informaticists.

Medola et al. (2018) report on the development of a customised low-cost upper limb prosthesis based on an interdisciplinary approach between researchers in product design and rehabilitation practitioners. They claim that such a collaboration is necessary because the rehabilitation professionals can focus on the user while the designers can focus on the product. Da Silva et al. (2019) report on the development of a customised transradial mechanical prosthesis for a patient with bilateral transradial amputation. They position the design process as interdisciplinary, combining the expertise of product designers and clinicians. The clinicians assessed the patient's characteristics, functional abilities and needs while the product designers focused on ergonomics and rapid prototyping. Olivares et al. (2020, p. 436) detail the set-up of an interdisciplinary collaboration established between computer scientists and occupational therapists specialised in traumatic brain injury (TBI) rehabilitation in order to design a technology that enhances the ability of individuals with severe cognitive impairments to complete a complex everyday activity such as preparing a hot meal. They offer the following justification for such a collaboration:

> On their own, computer scientists cannot apprehend a clientele as complex as TBI. They must work in partnership with clinical specialists who have developed, over the years, knowledge and experience in assisting this clientele on a daily basis. The design of assistive technologies specifically dedicated to TBI can only be interdisciplinary and intersectoral as fields as far apart as computer sciences and health must work collaboratively.

Understanding Interdisciplinarity as Multistakeholder Collaboration

Another core of AT research understands interdisciplinarity as multistakeholder collaboration that extends beyond the collaboration of academics and practitioners to include service providers, government agencies, policy makers, industrial partners and users. Smith and Boger (2022) argue that because AT provision is an interdisciplinary effort that includes end-users, interdisciplinary AT research should also include users. It is their contention that such an approach would increase the innovation of designs as well as the likelihood of real-world implementation. Examples of such research include Croxall et al. (2020) and Anvari et al. (2021).

Croxall et al. (2020) describe research that used qualitative methods to investigate the barriers to and facilitators of cultural participation for First Nations elders who use wheeled mobility and live on a reserve in Ontario, Canada. They label the research as interdisciplinary in nature because it engaged the perspectives of members of the First Nations community, care employees, policy analysts, academics, health advocacy officers and physiotherapists. Two key advantages of such an approach that Croxall et al. identified were the ability to increase the reach of dissemination and ensuring that the results were culturally relevant and usable.

Anvari et al. (2021) outline a programme of research that aimed to improve usability of an environmental control unit (ECU) interface for ex-members of the armed forces in the United States. The programme is defined as interdisciplinary, involving two academics with expertise in art, graphic design, engineering and human factors psychology; a government-funded rehabilitation centre for spinal cord injuries; and an industrial partner who manufactured ECUs. They claim that having an industrial partner strengthened the project by keeping it focused on realistic expectations for the outcome, while the government partner facilitated access to end-users, rehabilitation practitioners and home-care givers. Overall they conclude that the interdisciplinary nature of the project helped to increase the speed at which they could test ideas and get feedback.

A Call for More Transdisciplinary AT Research

The AT research and practice field makes no explicit distinctions between problem-focused and discipline-focused interdisciplinary research. However, there is a growing body of AT researchers who are calling for a kind of research that is capable of addressing complex problems that require innovative holistic solutions. They position this research as transdisciplinary rather than interdisciplinary. In addition to tackling complex problems (e.g., digital inequalities or capturing and evaluating AT outcomes), transdisciplinary AT research is situated as a collaborative endeavour involving academic and non-academic stakeholders (including AT users) that brings about transformational change (Grigorovich et al., 2019; Boger et al., 2017) Boger et al. (2017, p. 481) label complex problems as "wicked problems" that have no obvious apriori solution when teams begin their collaboration. They claim that:

> The ability to tackle wicked problems is essential in the development of assistive technologies since the experiential knowledge of the target population(s), professional knowledge of service providers and other stakeholders, and socio-scientific as well as humanistic knowledge must come together to address difficult, unstructured problems by re-thinking, re-working, and co-producing future possibilities.

Writing in the context of ageing and technology, Grigorovich et al. (2019) stress that the kind of collaboration that is required in transdisciplinary research is one that seeks to come to a consensus and focuses on achieving impact through, for example, changes in health outcomes, market adoption of technologies or changes in policy and/or practice.

Barriers to successful collaboration in interdisciplinary or transdisciplinary multistakeholder teams

Whether the research is interdisciplinary or transdisciplinary, there appears to be some agreement in the field that AT researchers need to engage in more collaborative research partnerships with a wider range of stakeholders, including users. Multistakeholder collaboration, however, is not easy. For example, Tait and Lyall (2007) document a range of problems that are experienced by interdisciplinary researchers such as language and communication issues and divergences in 'worldviews' across the disciplines. Difficulties such as these mean that more effort and time is required to make a success of a multistakeholder, collaborative research project. These difficulties are also experienced in AT research. For example, as part of their description of an interdisciplinary approach to developing an assistive upper limb exoskeleton for users with severe to complete functional tetraplegia, Struijk et al. (2022) report that it took a longer time to start up the project. Two reasons for this included differences in languages and expectations. Two examples of language differences offered by Struijk et al. (2022) involved the use of the words 'implementation' and 'case'. For clinicians, implementation meant using the technology in a clinical setting. For the engineers, implementation meant developing a new technical device. For the researchers, a case was understood as a project example. For the engineers, a case was interpreted as an application of a specific technology. With regards to differences in expectations, Struijk et al. (2022, p. 4) write: "We had different expectations for the user involvement; for the […] researchers, a deeper understanding of the users' lifeworld was important, while for the engineers, it related more to a joint brainstorming and feedback process on the exoskeleton use and design together with the users."

It would seem that two major barriers to multistakeholder collaboration within the field of disability and technology are lack of a common language and shared methods. Drawing on the ideas of Wenger (1998), it would seem that the various stakeholders have not yet been able to form a *community of practice*. In the next section I will expand on the community of practice theory to consider how it might be implemented in order to build the capacity of the AT research community to conduct interdisciplinary or transdisciplinary research.

Building Capacity to Conduct Interdisciplinary or Transdisciplinary Research by Building a Community of Practice

Definitions of communities of practice, offered by Beverley and Etienne Traynor-Wenger, suggest that there are commonalities between communities of practice and interdisciplinary or transdisciplinary research teams. Both involve collaboration, problem-solving and bringing about some kind of change:

> Communities of practice are sustained learning partnerships among people who share a concern or a passion for something they do and learn how to do it better as they interact regularly. Communities of practice also innovate and solve problems. They invent new practices, create new knowledge, define new territory and develop a collective and strategic voice.[2]

Communities of practice are essentially vehicles for learning (i.e., building capacity), and it is my contention that the disability and technology community needs to become a community of practice in order to learn how to conduct effective interdisciplinary or transdisciplinary research that solves the complex problems of digital inequality and inaccessibility.

Learning as a social process within a community of practice

Learning takes place in a community of practice through active participation in the group and is primarily a social process. A historical example of how a diverse group of stakeholders formed a successful community of practice, built on learning through social networking, is the case of the Special Education Microelectronic Resource Centres (SEMERCs) in the United Kingdom.

In 1982, the government in the United Kingdom created a centrally funded support network of centres and advisors for special education teachers (see Seale, 2022 for a more detailed account). The overarching aim of this network of centres and advisory teachers was to promote the use of microelectronics in the education of children with special educational needs and to provide a focal point for AT practice and research. At the core of the network were four regional SEMERCs and two Aids to Communication (ACE) Centres. Teachers could visit the SEMERCs in order to try out the latest hardware and software and access a national database of information about software. The SEMERCs also offered a series of newsletters, briefings, information sheets and training courses. In addition to providing resources and training, the ACE Centres assessed children referred by the local education authorities for their AT needs. The overarching strategy of this initiative for building the capacity of practitioners in the special education field was two-fold. Firstly, central funds were provided to enable local education authorities to second teachers to technology and special education advisory roles. These advisors would cascade what they had learnt from attending centre-led events back to their own schools and also support teachers within these schools to develop their use of technology in the classrooms. Secondly, a network of contacts with teachers and other professionals was built up and this network was used to facilitate multistakeholder meetings with practitioners, researchers and developers where participants could network, share ideas and contribute to developments in new AT.

Within the disability and technology field there are a number of networks that have similar aims to the SEMERCs (e.g., AAATE). While many of these networks comprise a variety of stakeholders, their foundations and histories are strongly rooted in one discipline or profession, typically rehabilitation and/ or rehabilitation engineering. This dominance (whether actual or perceived) of one particular discipline or stakeholder could be a significant barrier to the development of new interdisciplinary or transdisciplinary research practices in which all contributing stakeholders contribute on an equal or democratic basis. I would argue therefore that in order to build capacity for interdisciplinary and transdisciplinary AT research, a new network probably needs to be formed which creates its own history and traditions as it develops.

Sources of coherence for a community of practice

According to Wenger (1998), practice (e.g., interdisciplinary or transdisciplinary AT research) becomes a source of coherence for a community through mutual engagement, a joint enterprise and a shared repertoire.

People who want to participate in a community of practice are prepared to share their knowledge, improve their expertise, build up interpersonal networks and pursue their interest. This cannot be done by an individual in isolation from others. *Mutual engagement* requires responses from others and for these responses to lead to a continued engagement over time. A community of practice therefore cannot be formed from a one-off interaction (e.g., attending just one AT research related event, such as a conference or summit). If the disability and technology community wants to become an interdisciplinary/transdisciplinary community it will need to create and sustain a range of networking opportunities that engage all of its diverse stakeholders. For example, setting up a national or international exchange or secondment scheme, whereby members of one community (e.g., AT users) join another community (e.g., AT companies) for a period of time in order to share expertise and knowledge.

The practice of a community is shaped by its negotiated response to the conditions, resources and demands that members face. This negotiated response becomes a *joint enterprise*. In the context of AT research, the conditions could be the digital inequalities that AT users experience through lack of access to and inaccessibility of technologies. In terms of resources, the disability and technology community has to negotiate unpredictable funding levels for AT design, evaluation and provision. Demands that require a negotiated response from the community include mandates from policy makers for cost-effective AT solutions or for evidence of the outcomes of AT provision. If the disability and technology community wants to become an interdisciplinary or transdisciplinary community it will need to negotiate how to resource the collaboration of a large group of stakeholders and the time it takes to develop new shared ways of thinking and working.

A *shared repertoire* is the routines, words, tools, ways of doing things, stories, gestures, symbols, genres, actions or concepts that a community has produced or adopted in the course of its existence, and which have become part of its practice. At the moment, the AT research community has a shared repertoire that includes procedures to advise designers on what to do (e.g., Universal Design principles or Web Content Accessibility Guidelines); tools that enable members to perform an action (e.g., AT outcome measures such as the Quebec User Evaluation of Satisfaction with Assistive Technology); and laws or policies that enable members to make a case for action (e.g., United Nations Convention of the Rights of People with Disabilities). However, if the disability and technology community wants to become an interdisciplinary or transdisciplinary community, it will need to develop a shared repertoire to explicitly underpin its interdisciplinary/transdisciplinary practice. A starting point would be to come to a consensus about how to define interdisciplinary and transdisciplinary research in the field. The majority of members of the community are familiar with the ubiquitous definition of AT as an 'umbrella term for assistive products and their related systems and services'. We need them to also be able to find and implement a widely agreed definition of inter-disciplinary and transdisciplinary research. If the community agrees that the three variations of interdisciplinary research that I have identified earlier in this chapter each have a place, it would be useful to outline the circumstances (e.g., target grand challenge, intended outcomes) under which it would be appropriate to implement each one.

A constellation of practices

Wenger (1998) proposes that when a number of different communities of practice have related enterprises, face similar conditions, have members in common and share artefacts, they can be seen to form a *constellation*. With this in mind, I would contend that the disability and technology community is actually a constellation of different communities comprising AT users, AT policy makers, AT academics researchers, AT service providers, AT companies and AT research funders (see Figure 10.1).

When the communities within a constellation share artefacts, these can become *boundary objects*, a source of connection between communities. For example, I would suggest that the list of six grand challenges for AT outcomes produced by the Global Alliance of Assistive Technology Organisations (2022) has the potential to become a boundary object for AT policy makers, users, practi-tioners and researchers as they draw on the list and the work underpinning it to address key gaps in AT research and practice. We need similar artefacts which have been developed by all the communities within the constellation that set out what interdisciplinary/transdisciplinary AT research is and offer a set of guidance and case studies on what effective or 'best' interdisciplinary/transdisciplinary AT research looks like.

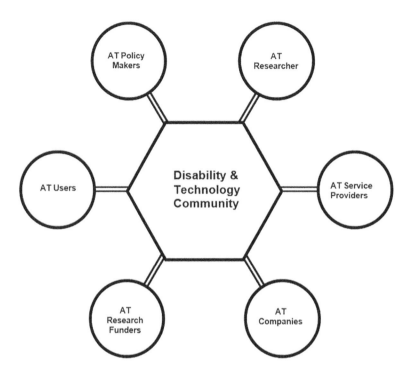

Figure 10.1   A constellation of AT communities of practice

Wenger argued that when people transfer from one community of practice to another, or have multi-membership, they can transfer some element of one practice into another through brokering. Wenger labels such people as *brokers*. Brokers are able to make new connections across communities of practice. They enable coordination and open new possibilities for meaning. It is through these connections that new interdisciplinary or transdisciplinary research practices can develop. It may be helpful therefore for the disability and technology community to consider whether there are existing roles within the community that might be best suited to brokering such connections between different connected communities, or whether new roles need to be created, like the special advisory teacher roles that were created as part of the SEMERC initiative that I described earlier in this chapter. It may also be useful to debate whether there is a need to teach 'brokering' skills in AT professional education and development courses such as the MSc in Educational Assistive Technology described in Chapter 8.

Conclusion

The field of disability and technology is a 'broad church' comprising many different disciplines, professionals and stakeholders. The breadth of the field has the potential to be a great strength if all those in the different communities can work together sufficiently well to develop a shared history and understanding of how best to conduct collaborative interdisciplinary or transdisciplinary research that will address the grand research challenges of the future.

Notes

1   AAATE 2023 Conference Programme. https://aaate2023.eu/wp-content/uploads/sites/26/2023/08/AAATE2023-Programme.pdf
2   https://www.wenger-trayner.com/communities-of-practice/

References

Aboelela, S.W., Larson, E., Bakken S., Carrasquillo, O., Formicola, A., Glied, S.A., Haas, J., & Gebbie, K.M. (2007). Defining interdisciplinary research: Conclusions from a critical review of the literature. *Health Service Research*, *42*(1), 329–46. DOI:10.1111/j.1475–6773.2006.00621.x

Anvari, S.S., Hancock, G.M., Mok, N.B., Ayvazyan, A., Macado, C.L., Chompff, R.M.E., McCoy, K.M., Nare, M.T., Shiraiwa, Y., Mizushima, Y., Morales, N., & Acharbaji, L. (2021). Interface Design for Users with Spinal Cord Injuries and Disorders: An Interdisciplinary Research Program with the US Department of Veterans Affairs. In N.L. Black, W.P. Neumann, & I. Noy (Eds.), *Proceedings of the 21st Congress of the International Ergonomics Association (IEA 2021). Lecture Notes in Networks and Systems. vol 222.* (pp. 232–238). Springer. https://doi.org/10.1007/978-3-030-74611-7_32

Boger, J., Jackson, P., Mulvenna, M., Sixsmith, J., Sixsmith, A., Mihailidis, A., Kontos, P., Polgar, J.M., Grigorovich, A., & Martin, S. (2017). Principles for fostering the transdisciplinary development of assistive technologies. *Disability and Rehabilitation: Assistive Technology*, *12*(5), 480–490. DOI:10.3109/17483107.2016.1151953

Cheng, J.L.C., Henisz, W.J., Roth, K., & Swaminathan, A. (2009). From the editors: Advancing interdisciplinary research in the field of international business: Prospects, issues and challenges. *Journal of International Business Studies, 40*, 1070–1074.

Croxall, L., Gifford, W., & Jutai, J. (2020). First Nations elders who use wheeled mobility: An exploration of culture and health. *Canadian Journal on Aging, 39*(2), 318–327. DOI:10.1017/S0714980819000655

Da Silva, L.A., Medola, F.O., Rodrigues, O.V., Rodrigues, A.C.T., & Sandnes, F.E. (2019). Interdisciplinary-based Development of User-friendly Customized 3D Printed Upper Limb Prosthesis. In T. Ahram & C. Falcão (Eds.), *Advances in Usability, User Experience and Assistive Technology. AHFE 2018. Advances in Intelligent Systems and Computing.* vol 794, (pp. 899–908). Springer. https://doi.org/10.1007/978-3-319-94947-5_88

Global Alliance of Assistive Technology Organisations (2022). *GAATO AT Outcomes Grand Challenge Consultation.* https://www.gaato.org/grand-challenges

Griffin, G., Medhurst., P. & Green, T. (2006). *Interdisciplinarity in Interdisciplinary Research Programmes in the UK.* University of Hull. Available from: https://www.researchgate.net/profile/Gabriele-Griffin/publication/254357611_Interdisciplinary_Research_Programmes_in_the_UK/links/5515b17f0cf2f7d80a34aeaa/Interdisciplinary-Research-Programmes-in-the-UK.pdf

Grigorovich, A., Fang, M.L., Sixsmith, J., & Kontos, P. (2019). Defining and evaluating transdisciplinary research: Implications for aging and technology. *Disability and Rehabilitation: Assistive Technology, 14*(6), 533–542. DOI:10.1080/17483107.2018.1496361

Haltaufderheide, J., Hovemann, J., & Vollmann, J. (Eds.) (2020). *Aging between Participation and Simulation.* Gruyter. https://doi.org/10.1515/9783110677485

Institute of Medicine (2005). *Facilitating Interdisciplinary Research.* The National Academies Press. https://doi.org/10.17226/11153

Klein, J.T., & Newell, W.H. (1997). Advancing interdisciplinary studies. In J.G. Gaff & J.L. Ratcliff (Eds.), *Handbook of the Undergraduate Curriculum: A Comprehensive Guide to Purposes, Structures, Practices, and Change* (pp. 393–415). Jossey-Bass.

Koumpouros, Y. (2021). A highly user-centered design approach for developing a mobile health app for pain management (PainApp). *Proceedings of the 14th Pervasive Technologies Related to Assistive Environments Conference* (pp. 320–329). https://doi.org/10.1145/3453892.3461350

Medola, F.O., Sandnes, F.E., da Silva, S.R., & Rodrigues, A.C. (2018). Improving assistive technology in practice: Contributions from interdisciplinary research and development collaboration. *Assistive Technology Outcomes and Benefits, 12*(1), 1–10.

Olivares, M., Pigot, H., Bottari, C., Lavoie, M., Zayani, T., Bier, N., Le Dorze, G., Pinard, S., Le Pevedic, B., Swaine, B., Therriault, P-Y., Thépaut, A., & Giroux, S. (2020). Use of a persona to support the interdisciplinary design of an assistive technology for meal preparation in traumatic brain injury. *Interacting with Computers, 32*(5–6), 435–456. https://doi.org/10.1093/iwcomp/iwab002

Pascher, M., Baumeister, A., Schneegass, S., Klein, B., & Gerken, J. (2021). Recommendations for the Development of a Robotic Drinking and Eating Aid – An Ethnographic Study. In C. Ardito., R. Lanzilotti., A. Malizioa, H. Petrie, A. Piccinno, G. Desolda, & K. Inkpen (Eds.), *Human-Computer Interaction-INTERACT 2021. Lecture Notes in Computer Science, 12932* (pp. 331–351). Springer. https://doi.org/10.1007/978-3-030-85623-6_21

Plattner, J., Oberrauner, E., Ströckl, D.E., & Oberzaucher, J. (2020). Using IoT middleware solutions in interdisciplinary research projects in the context of AAL. *Proceedings of the 13th ACM International Conference on Pervasive Technologies Related to Assistive Environments (PETRA '20).* (Article 51, pp. 1–6). Association for Computing Machinery. https://doi.org/10.1145/3389189.3397986

Schulz, R., Wahl, H.-W., Matthews, J.T., De Vito Dabbs, A., Beach, S.R., & Czaja, S.J. (2015). Advancing the aging and technology agenda in gerontology. *The Gerontologist, 55,* 724–734.

Schwaninger, I., Güldenpfennig, F., Weiss, A., & Fitzpatrick, G. (2021). What Do You Mean by Trust? Establishing Shared Meaning in Interdisciplinary Design for Assistive Technology. *International Journal of Social Robotics, 13,* 1879–1897. https://doi.org/10.1007/s12369-020-00742-w

Seale, J. (2022). *Technology Use by Adults with Learning Disabilities Past, Present and Future Design and Support Practices.* Routledge

Shaw, S., Bernardi, F., & Nickpour, F. (2022). Child-centred framing through design research: A framework for analysing children's 'dream wheelchair' designs to elicit meaning and elevate their voice. *Disability and Rehabilitation: Assistive Technology,* DOI:10.1080/17483107.2022.2071487

Smith, E.M., & Boger, J. (2022). Better together: Promoting interdisciplinary research in assistive technology. *Assistive Technology, 34*(1), 1–1. DOI:10.1080/10400435.2022.2047397

Struijk, L.N.S.A., Kanstrup, A.M., Bai, S., Bak, T., Thogersen, M.B., Mohammadi, M., Bengtson, S.H., Kobbelgaard, F.V., Gull, M.A., Bentsen, B., Severinsen, K.E., Kasch, H., & Moeslund, T.B. (2022). The impact of interdisciplinarity and user involvement on the design and usability of an assistive upper limb exoskeleton – a case study on the EXOTIC. *Proceedings of the International Conference on Rehabilitation Robotics* (pp. 1–5). IEEE. https://doi.org/10.1109/ICORR55369.2022.9896500

Tait, J., & Lyall, C. (2007). *Short Guide to Developing Interdisciplinary Research Proposals.* The Institute for The Study of Science Technology and Innovation (ISSTI) Briefing Note, Number 1 (March). https://jlesc.github.io/downloads/docs/ISSTI _Briefing_Note_1-Writing_Interdisciplinary_Research_Proposals.pdf

Van den Heuvel, R., Jansels, R., Littler, B., Huijnen, C., Di Nuovo, A., Bonarini, A., Lorenzo, D., Encarnação, P., Lekova, A., & de Witte, L. (2022). The potential of robotics for the development and wellbeing of children with disabilities as we see it. *Technology and Disability, 34*(1), 25–33. DOI:10.3233/TAD-210346

Wenger, E. (1998). *Communities of Practice: Learning, Meaning and Identity.* Cambridge University Press.

WHO & UNICEF (2022). *Global Report on Assistive Technology.* https://apps.who.int/iris/handle/10665/354357

Index